THE SEX BIBLE

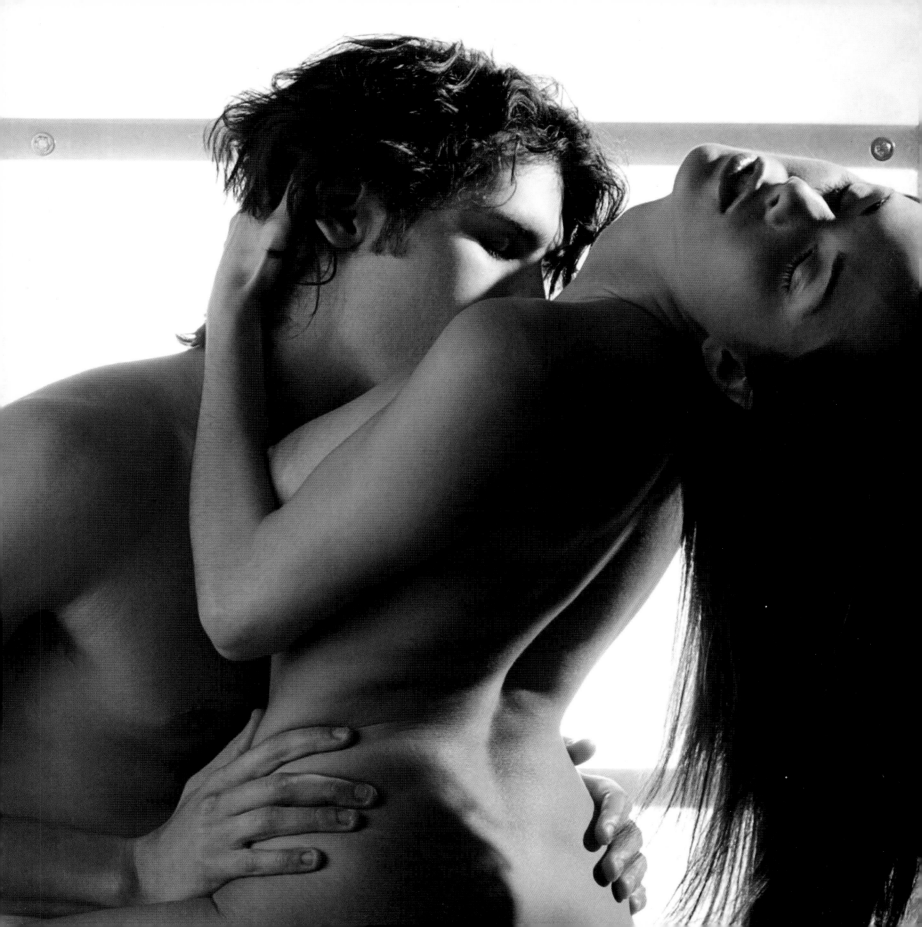

THE
SEX

**THE COMPLETE GUIDE
TO SEXUAL LOVE**

BIBLE

Susan Crain Bakos

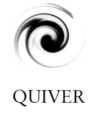

QUIVER

DEDICATION

This book is for Hugh Hunte,
who could talk me through anything.

May you never lose your voice, darlin'.

Text © 2006 by Susan Crain Bakos
Photography © 2006 Rockport Publishers
This paperback edition first published in 2008

First published in the USA in 2006 by
Quiver, a member of
Quayside Publishing Group
100 Cummings Center
Suite 406-L
Beverly, MA 01915-6101
www.quiverbooks.com

The publisher maintains the records relating to images in this book required by 18 USC 2257 which
records are located at Rockport Publishers, Inc. 100 Cummings Center, Suite 406-L, Beverly MA 01915

10 09 08   1 2 3 4 5

ISBN - 13: 978-1-59233-285-4
ISBN - 10: 1-59233-285-4

Library of Congress Cataloging-in-Publication Data
Bakos, Susan Crain.
    The sex bible : the complete guide to sensual love / Susan Crain Bakos. -- 1st U.S. ed.
        p. cm.
    ISBN-13: 978-1-59233-227-4 (Hardcover)
    1. Sex instruction. 2. Sex. I. Title.
    HQ31.B23497 2006
    613.9'6--dc22

                                                                    2006012109

Cover design by Loewy: London: www.loewygroup.com
Book design by Carol Holtz Design
Photography by Allan Penn
Photos on page 205 reprinted with permission of Good Vibrations.

Printed and bound in Singapore

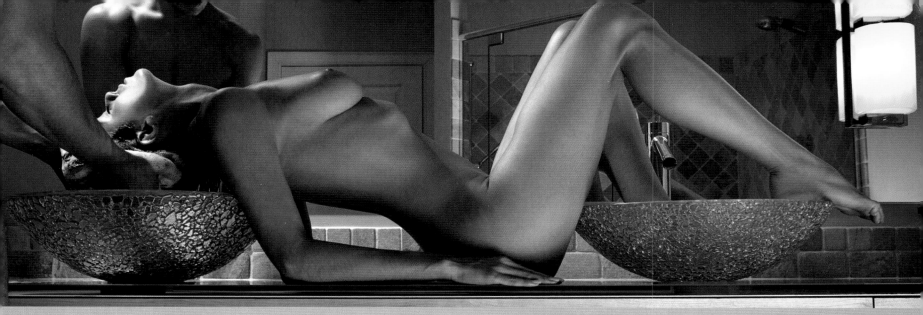

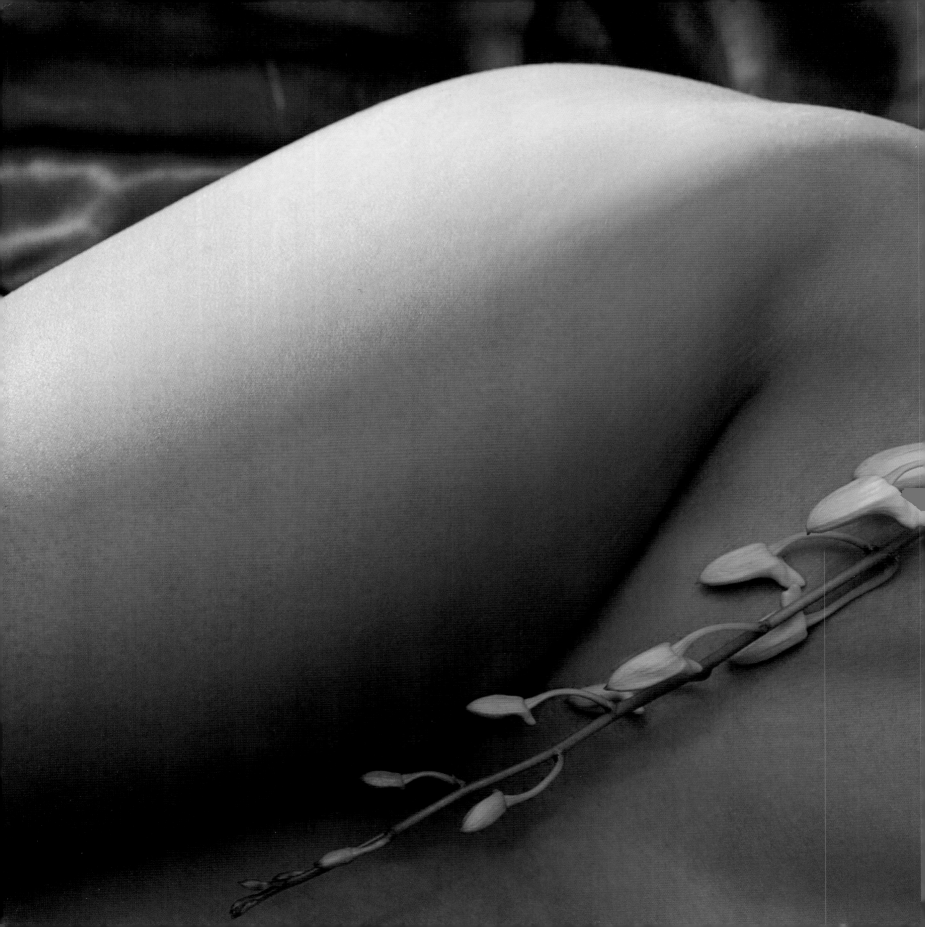

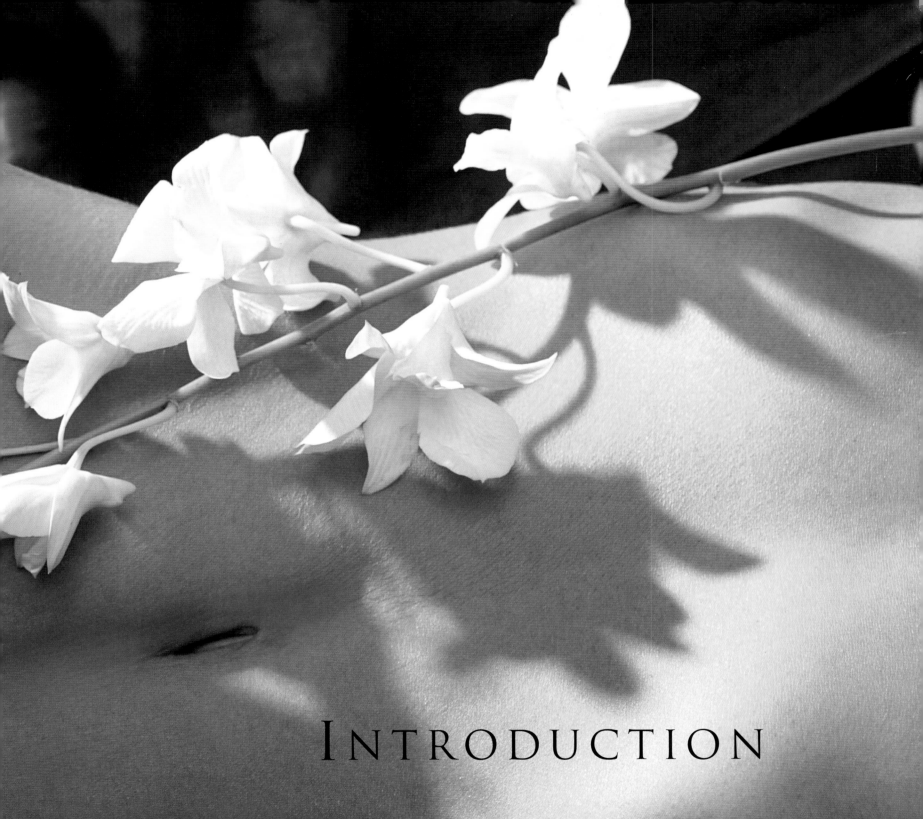

INTRODUCTION

WHAT I REALLY KNOW
TO BE SEXUALLY TRUE

___

OPRAH WINFREY HAS a favorite question she asks celebrities and others: "What do you really know to be true?"

It's a good question. We too often accept "truths" without checking their validity. The Internet has only exacerbated the situation.

As a journalist, I've discovered that the "facts" repeated over and over again in magazine articles and books are sometimes not quite true—and occasionally blatantly false. For more than two decades, sex has been my area of journalistic expertise. When the subject is sex, the information presented as true is often slanted to satisfy what an editor thinks the readers want to read. So for years we read that "intimacy" is more important to women than orgasms, that "communicating feelings" is a more valuable lovemaking skill than sex technique— and that men don't call because they're terrified of the tremendous love/desire they feel for us. (Oh, ha, ha, ha!) There are still some women's service magazines where masturbation is a taboo subject—and the best-selling book *He's Just Not That Into You* (in which a man tells women exactly why men don't call and a few other things) hasn't penetrated the collective staff consciousness. It may as well be 1959.

If a woman has never masturbated, how likely is it that she knows *how* she reaches orgasm? Not very. She's depending on her partner and serendipity to get her there—when the truth would set her free.

Unlike most sex journalists and therapist/authors, I've been "test-driving" the techniques I write about for twenty years.

I have also asked hundreds of women (and men) to test techniques and report back to me for magazine articles and books. I am the author of six sex advice books—including the international best-seller *Sexational Secrets: "The Ultimate Guide to Erotic Know-How."* I approach sex writing with a spirit of scientific inquiry. In researching those books I have studied sex technique with Tantric and Taoist masters, porn stars and directors, great therapists such as Dr. Ruth Westheimer and the late Dr. Helen Singer Kaplan, sexual innovators such as Annie Sprinkle—and many others.

What I learned to be true: The problematic nature of female orgasm is the big engine driving every sex philosophy, therapy, and theory.

Many women experience difficulty in reaching orgasm—with a partner, during intercourse, or simply as often as they would like. Their problem: getting distracted from arousal by body or performance anxiety, guilt over work/chores/children, anger or resentment against the partner—and getting so distracted that reaching orgasm "takes too long" and consequently doesn't always happen. In other words, most women just don't focus on sex in the single-minded way that men do.

Male sexuality is awesome in its single-minded power.

A FEW YEARS AGO, I began tinkering with orgasm techniques based on my own research and that of others, especially the cognitive feedback studies of Dr. Eileen Palace in New Orleans. Using my love of art, I developed the concept of a sensual and beautiful arousal image, an image that a woman will always associate with her arousal, such as a Georgia O'Keefe flower print or even

WHAT I KNOW TO BE SEXUALLY TRUE:

- Women like sex better when they reach orgasm often— and that's not going to happen for most women without direct clitoral stimulation.

- Both men and women are more confident sexually if they have good technique.

- Men are more intimate—closely connected—in their relationships with women when the sex is good.

- And good sex smoothes our personal rough edges so that man and woman can live together in some kind of harmony. We need sex.

a color or a sunset over the ocean. I simplified and refined the breathing techniques I learned from Tantra teachers and applied the one basic trick every woman should have in her erotic kit: flexing the pubococcygeus muscle. But something was still missing. I did not yet have the works-every-time, absolutely fail-safe-once-you've-learned-it orgasm method for every woman.

An old friend in Illinois who has five black belts in karate taught me energy focus—the way he does it when he moves all the energy in his body, for example, into his throat to prevent an arrow from piercing his skin.

And that was the missing piece, the completing step of the Orgasm Loop. Arousal image, energy focus, physical techniques. It takes a little practice, like riding a bike, but once you've learned it, you do it automatically. And—wow!—does it work.

When I was offered the opportunity to write *The Sex Bible*, I was thrilled, because it was the chance to bring together what I have learned in twenty years of research-ing sex and interviewing men and women about their sex lives—*and* incorporate my own Orgasm Loop. In this book I tell you the best of what *I* know to be true and give you what *you* need to know to be a good, even great, lover. The beautiful erotic photographs—the best I have seen in a sex book—will inspire you. They are alive with erotic energy and infused with romance.

The Sex Bible is truly a beautiful book about the most intimate part of life. I am more proud of this book than of anything I've done, but I haven't created it alone. *The Sex Bible* is a team effort of three people: Allan Penn, the photographer; Wendy Gardner, the visionary force; and me.

I speak for all of us when I say, may it bring you pleasure.

Susan Crain Bakos
Harlem, New York City
February 2006

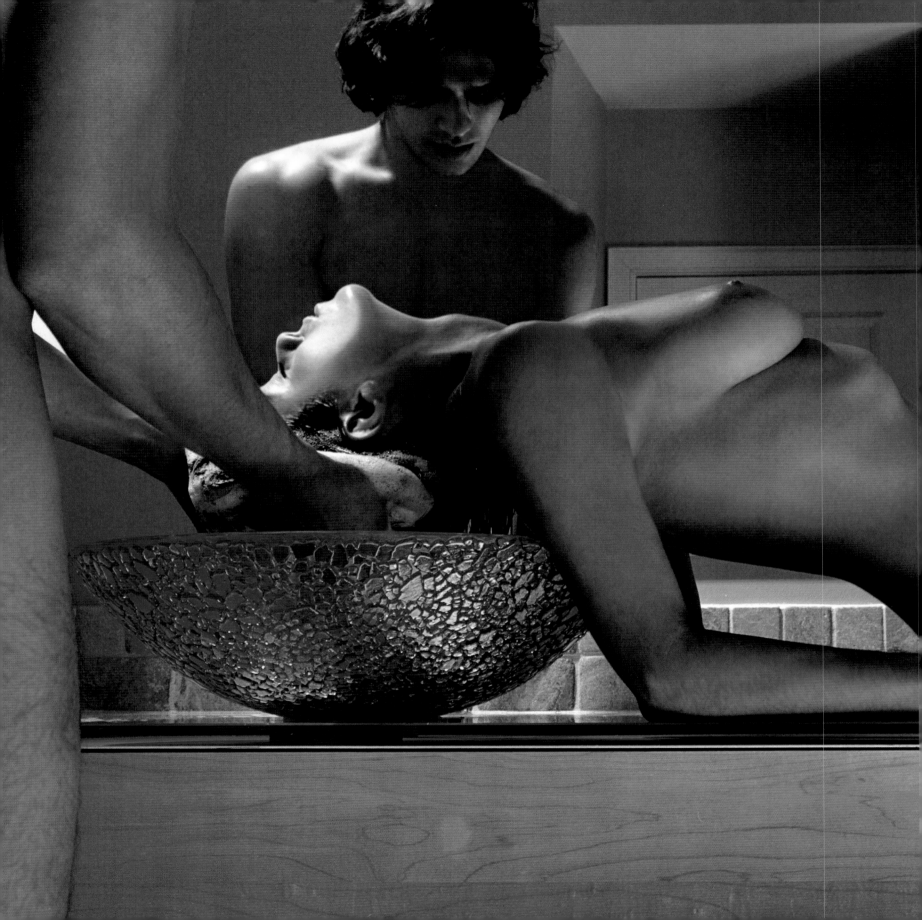

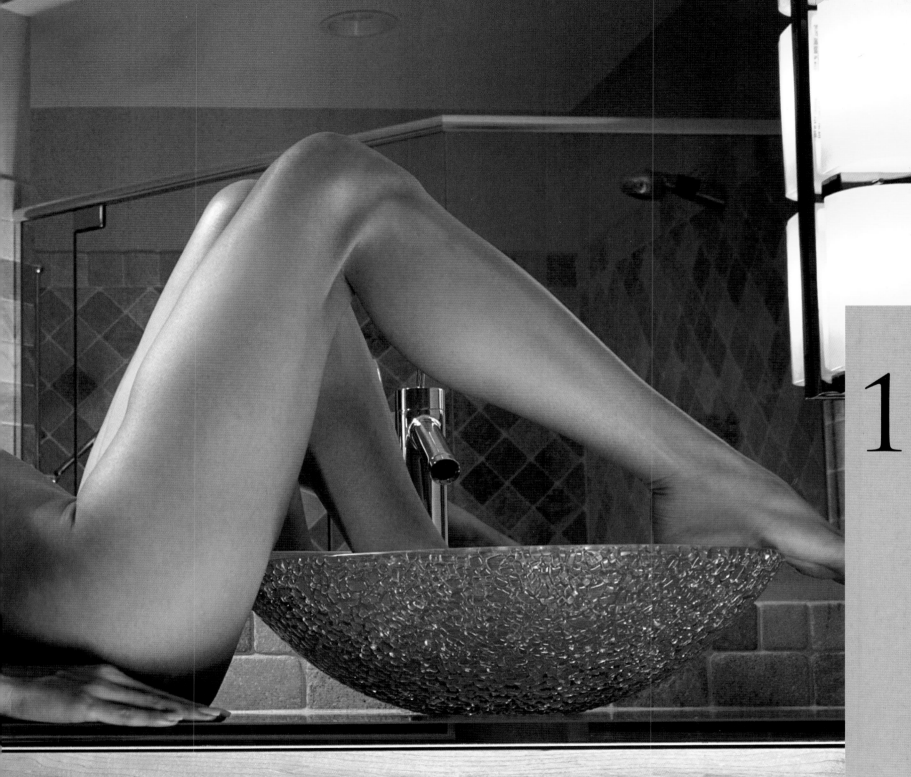

1

SEDUCTION

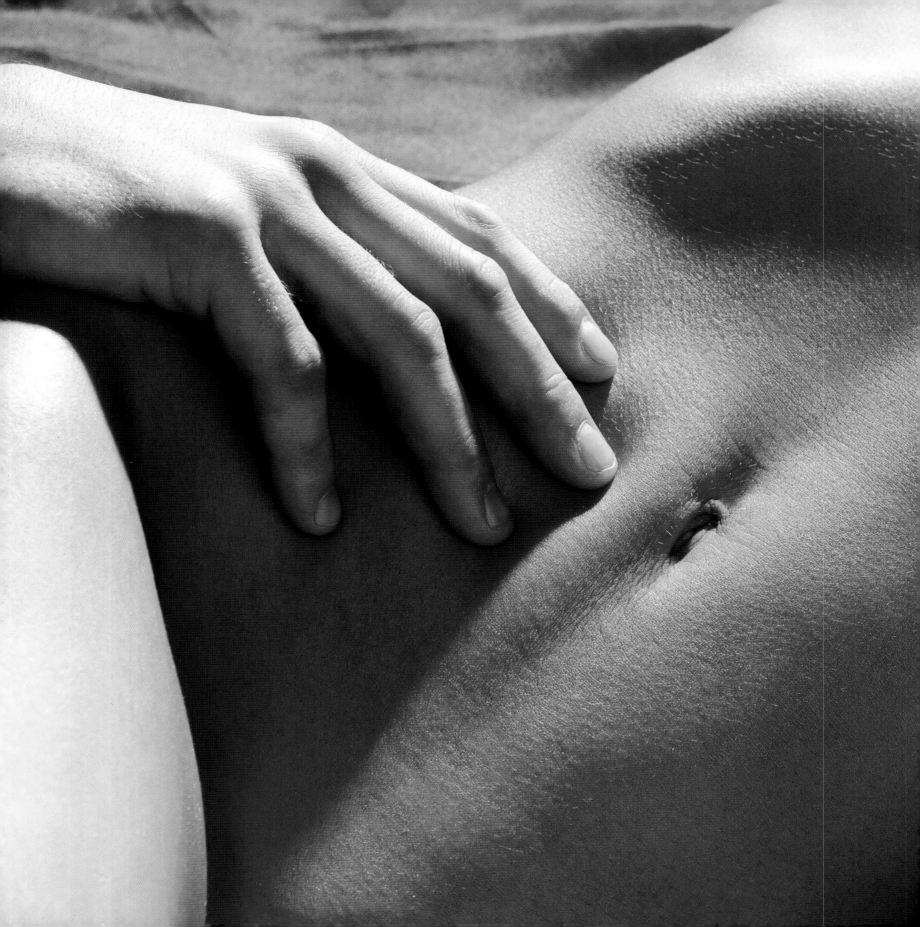

THE ARTFUL PATH
TO THE BEDROOM

———

"Seduction is always more singular

and sublime than sex."

— Jean Baudrillard
French philosopher

IN OTHER WORDS, the thrill of the sexual chase can be even more exciting than the lovemaking for some people. (If these people are men, we call them Casanovas or Don Juans.) For others, seduction is an intrinsic part of the sexual process, not more important than, but equal to, the joy of sex. Camille Paglia, an American philosopher, author, and critic known for her controversial essays on popular culture, takes this view.

She says, "Pursuit and seduction are the essence of sexuality. It's part of the sizzle."

Seduction is the indispensable opening act to great sex. But it's also a pleasurable pursuit that can stand on its own.

Seduction is a delicious game, more of the mind than of the body, which has been well played by courtesans and famous lovers throughout the centuries. From Cleopatra to Angelina Jolie, from Casanova to Mick Jagger, the great seducers could lure almost anyone into their beds. Not all great seducers were or are beautiful and handsome. Cleopatra, for example, had a big nose, a short waist—and bore no resemblance to Elizabeth Taylor, who, in her magnificent prime, played the Egyptian queen on screen. In spite of her physical shortcomings, Cleopatra—an intelligent, well-read woman who captivated men with her mind—held two of Rome's most powerful men, Julius Caesar and Mark Anthony, in her thrall.

Some people say they don't like to play games. They want to go straight to "the sex" and expect the object of their desires to hurry along with them. And they think that makes them somehow more "sincere" or "honest" than the rest of us!

"I just want to be me, no games" actually translates into "I don't want to put any effort into getting you into bed." The artless approach works sometimes—especially when the partners know each other very well and are both in need of a quickie. But in the beginning, and frequently thereafter, seducing your partner is a pleasure in itself and certainly makes "the sex" a richer and more satisfying experience. Furthermore, you may not get to the bedroom at all—or as often as you would like—if you don't know how to seduce.

It has been said that seduction is a lost art, gone with civilized conversation and dressing well for air travel, a casualty of a society that values frankness, speed, and function over form. Sexual, not sensual, imagery permeates our culture. And seduction celebrates sensuality, bringing the couple to their senses—all five of them. But a lost art? No.

A COUPLE'S STORY

Melanie met Andrew at a jazz festival the year they were both twenty-two. She thought he was handsome. He thought she was beautiful. Neither of them had the courage (or the seduction skills) to approach the other. But she fantasized about him, he about her. Luckily they ran into each other the following year at the same jazz festival.

"I had learned something about seducing a woman by then," Andrew says. "I wasn't going to let her get away this time."

He walked up to her and said, "I remember you from last year. I could never forget a woman as beautiful as you."

Melanie was flattered and responded warmly to his overture and told him, "I remember you, too."

"I've thought about you a lot," he said, his gaze locked into hers.

"And I've thought about you, too," she said, impulsively reaching out a hand to touch his arm.

With that touch, she seized opportunity. They have been together ever since.

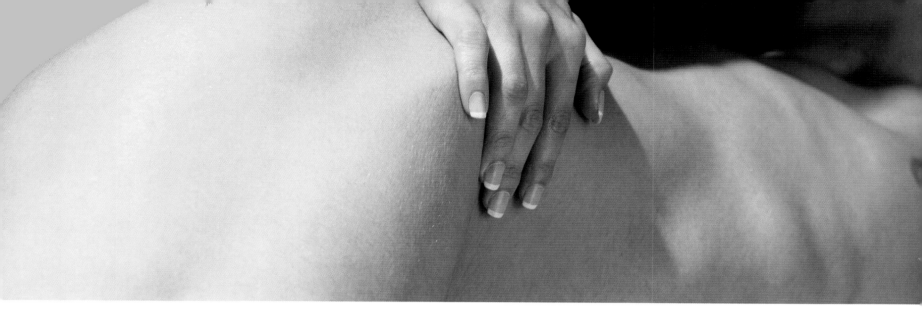

THE ELEMENTS
OF SEDUCTION

Flirting

Some people are born flirts. And that's a good thing. Flirting is a natural human instinct, practiced in all cultures and throughout history. Our puritanical society has given flirting a bad name, most recently under the guise of political correctness rules. Hardly a sin or a crime, flirting is essentially the ability to charm, a way of making both you and the object of your attentions feel more vibrantly, sexually alive.

Technique Tip

DRESS FOR IT

When you meet friends after work or go out alone, take the time to turn your day outfit into a nightworthy one, as you'd do if you had a date. Unfasten some buttons. Switch tops or shoes. Spray on a little fragrance. You never know whose senses you will want to awaken.

Meeting your husband or significant other? Dress for him—and flirt with him—just like you did when you were first dating.

OPENING LINES

Research shows that 55 percent of a first romantic impression is based on looks, 38 percent on speaking style, and a mere 7 percent on the words actually spoken. That explains why opening gambits such as "Haven't I seen you someplace before?" or "Some weather, huh?" ever do work. It's good news for the nervous, shy, and tongue-tied. You don't have to come up with something clever. In fact, "I've been admiring you from across the room" can seem brilliant.

But, if you can speak in coherent sentences in the presence of someone you desire, words can woo a certain kind of woman in a way that nothing else can.

> *"All really great lovers are articulate*
>
> *and verbal seduction*
>
> *is the surest road to actual seduction."*
>
> — Marya Mannes
> American journalist

Very intelligent women, and men, are seduced (though not exclusively) by words. You make contact with their bodies by connecting with their minds first. Remember Cleopatra.

EYE CONTACT

Flirting begins with the eyes.

Have you ever watched a couple connect at a crowded bar or party? They glance at each other—with ever so slightly raised eyebrows—look away, glance back, eventually holding the eye contact long enough to indicate mutual interest. If they don't make their way toward each other immediately, they will soon.

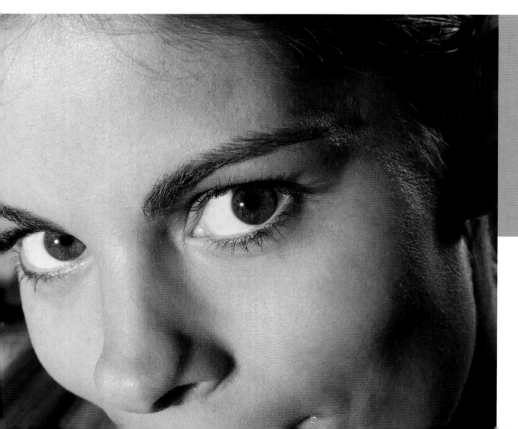

"Real talk"

"You can have an intimate conversation with a stranger just using your eyes," says Annie, a twenty-nine-year-old consummate flirt. "Think specifically sexy thoughts about him. Women can undress men with their eyes, too."

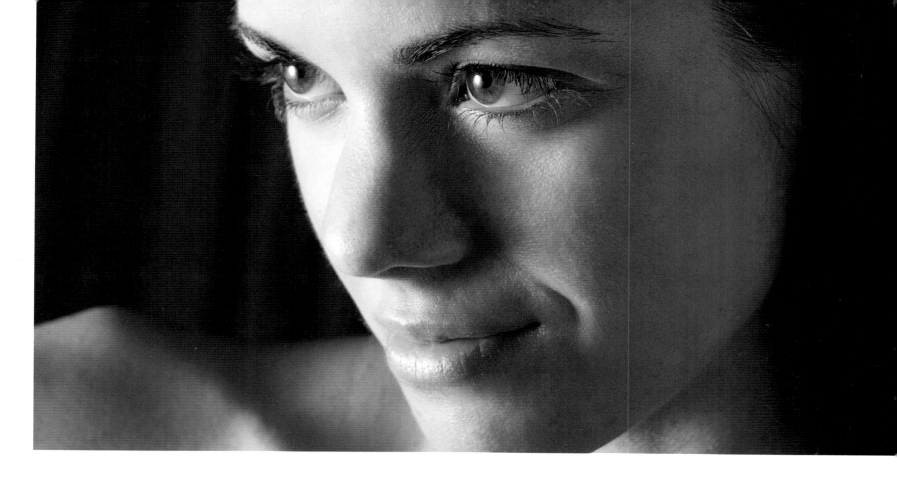

When a couple are close together, the eye flirting takes on another dimension. They look into each other's eyes, and then lower their gazes to include the mouths, raise back to the eyes again—and expand their gaze to include the body. A sweeping glance that takes in her cleavage and legs or his torso before returning to the eyes says, *I am attracted to you.*

Studies have also shown that women who are very attracted to a man blink more frequently than normal during eye contact with him. The phrase "batting her eyes" comes from that response. Princess Diana was famous for flirtatiously batting her eyes. In the classic posture, chin down, eyes up, she double-blinked and captivated just about every man in eye range except Prince Charles.

The "chin slightly down, eyes gazing slightly" position is key to the success of batting one's eyes. Do it while looking straight on at a man and you risk appearing silly at worst, immediately transparent at best.

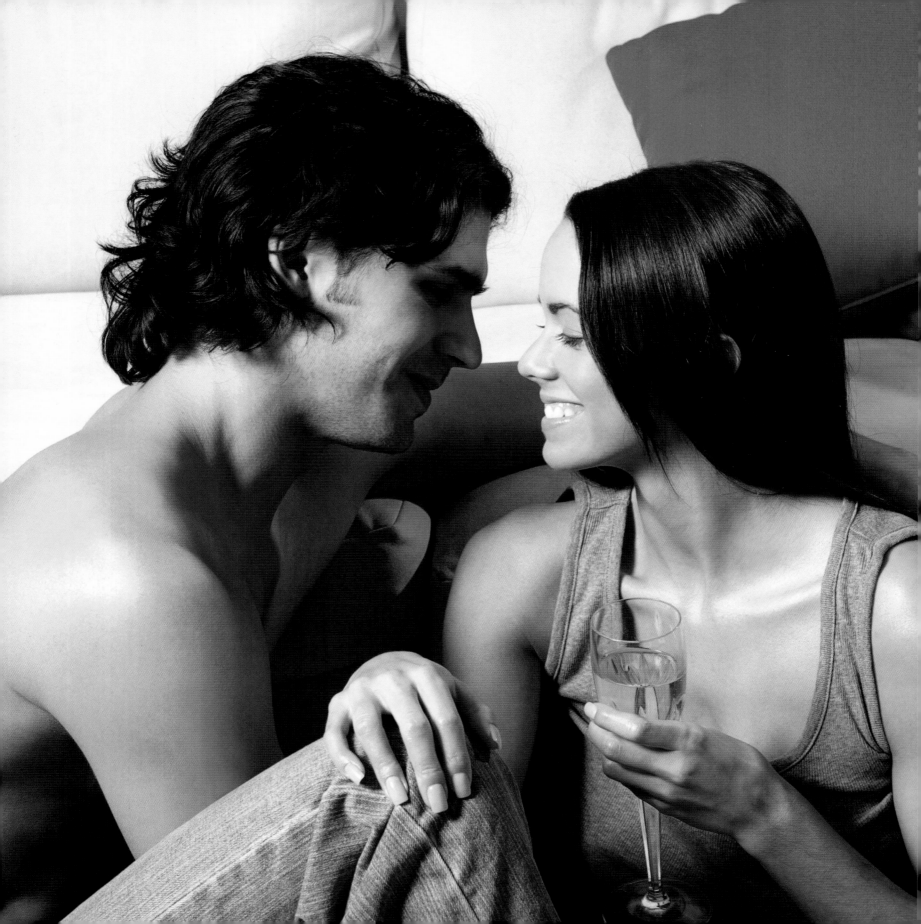

PHYSICAL GESTURES

The hair toss may be a movie cliché, but it is also a little seductive move commonly acted out on barstools every night of the week all over the world. When a woman tosses back long hair, twists a curl around her finger, or otherwise plays with her hair while talking to or gazing at a man, she's sending him one of the oldest signals a woman *can* send a man. Translation: *Hey, I am interested in you.* And it works because every man picks up that signal on a subliminal level.

If you've stopped flirting with your guy in this way, begin anew. Sometimes reviving flagging desire is as simple as paying attention to each other in that flirtatious way. It's highly unfortunate when couples lose the habit of flattering each other.

"Real talk"

"I like to flirt and do it a lot," says Annie. "But I learned to flirt selectively. If you really like a guy and he sees you treating all the guys the same way, he won't feel special. And he may not come on to you. So flirt a lot for practice if there's nobody you really want in the room, but focus on one guy when you want to make something happen. Men are really flattered by the attention."

Technique Tip

If you have short hair, running your fingers through your hair or otherwise fluffing it up sends the same message—as long as you are looking at him when you do it.

Most physical gestures, such as the hair toss, are unconscious. Think about them and make your movements more seductive. If you can do this comfortably, make a gesture that draws attention to one of your best features. For example, while conversing with someone else (but in his eyesight), run a finger abstractedly down your throat to the top of your breasts.

Or strike a *quick* pose for her. Make sure she sees your profile in the best light. You want these gestures to be obvious—yet so brief that the viewer can't be entirely sure they were meant to be seen.

Men often show their interest by "grooming" themselves for her. While looking at her, he might straighten his tie, smooth the front of his shirt, slick back an errant lock of hair. He's saying, *I want you to find me attractive.*

Both sexes may touch themselves in subtle (and nongenital!) ways. He may rest his hands on his strong thighs. She may cross and uncross her pretty legs, brushing her fingers against them as she pulls down her skirt. If the room is chilly, she crosses her arms and strokes them, ostensibly for warmth.

A COUPLE'S STORY

My grandmother was a world-class flirt," Kim says. "She charmed men to the end of her life at the age of ninety. I'm sure she never cheated on Grandpa, but she sure did remind him why he married her and that he wasn't the only one on line. She's my role model."

Kim and Josh, in their mid-thirties, have been together for ten years, married for six. They have an agreement that flirting with other people is acceptable. It's okay, for example, for her to bat her eyes and engage in sexual banter with a stranger at a party. And it's okay, for example, for him to make mischievous eye contact with another woman, touch her arm, and tell her how beautiful she is.

"Flirting occasionally with other people keeps our juices flowing," Josh says. "Remember that old line 'I'm married, not dead.' We see no harm and definite benefits from simple flirtation."

"Getting attention from another man makes me feel sexy," Kim says. "It reinforces all the good messages that Josh gives me. I'm always suspicious of people who say you can't flirt with anyone else once you're married. I think they may be more likely to have an affair than I am!"

Flirting in social situations has another benefit: They are inspired to flirt more with each other after "playing around" with others. In fact, a little public flirting is often the prelude to an intense seduction at home.

"It's like seduction foreplay," he explains. "We often leave a party or dinner engagement with friends where we've exercised our flirt muscles and can't keep our hands off each other in the car driving home. She plays with my thigh. I reach over and caress her breast at a stop sign. Stoplights give us time for a passionate kiss."

Are they ever jealous of each other?

"Occasionally," she says, "but only a little."

"I experience flashes of jealousy," he says, "but that adds to the experience. It makes me try harder with her."

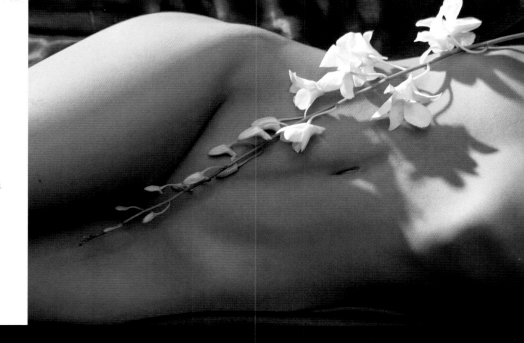

BODY LANGUAGE

"Attraction" or "courtship" body language is the universal language of would-be lovers. Typically the body dialogue is more obvious to observers than to the couple in full flirt mode. Hands and feet are pointed toward each other. If they are sitting together at a bar, his legs are open, hers closed and in the space between his, their bodies not touching. Whether standing or sitting, they lean, from the waist up, toward each other. Soon they are "mirroring" each other—that is, unconsciously copying gestures and expressions.

Essential Skills

Making a Woman (or a Man) Feel Sexy

A sexy Italian man noted for his appeal to women once said, "If you don't make a woman feel sexy, she is not going to bed with you."

Some men resort to the general compliment "You're beautiful." Maybe she is and maybe she isn't?but the generic compliment can fall flat. She will feel beautiful, however, if you notice what's really special about her and praise that. *You have the smoothest legs. Your hair is lovely. Has anyone ever told you that your eyes are beautiful?*

For a woman seducing a man, the advice needs to be phrased a little differently. Men feel emasculated when they are criticized or treated with even playful disdain in public. (Certainly that is not a state conducive to sex.) While banter might be part of seduction, assess his limits. Don't tease too hard. Too many couples do that to each other. Then they wonder why they "never" have sex.

Admire a man and you make him feel powerful—and sexy.

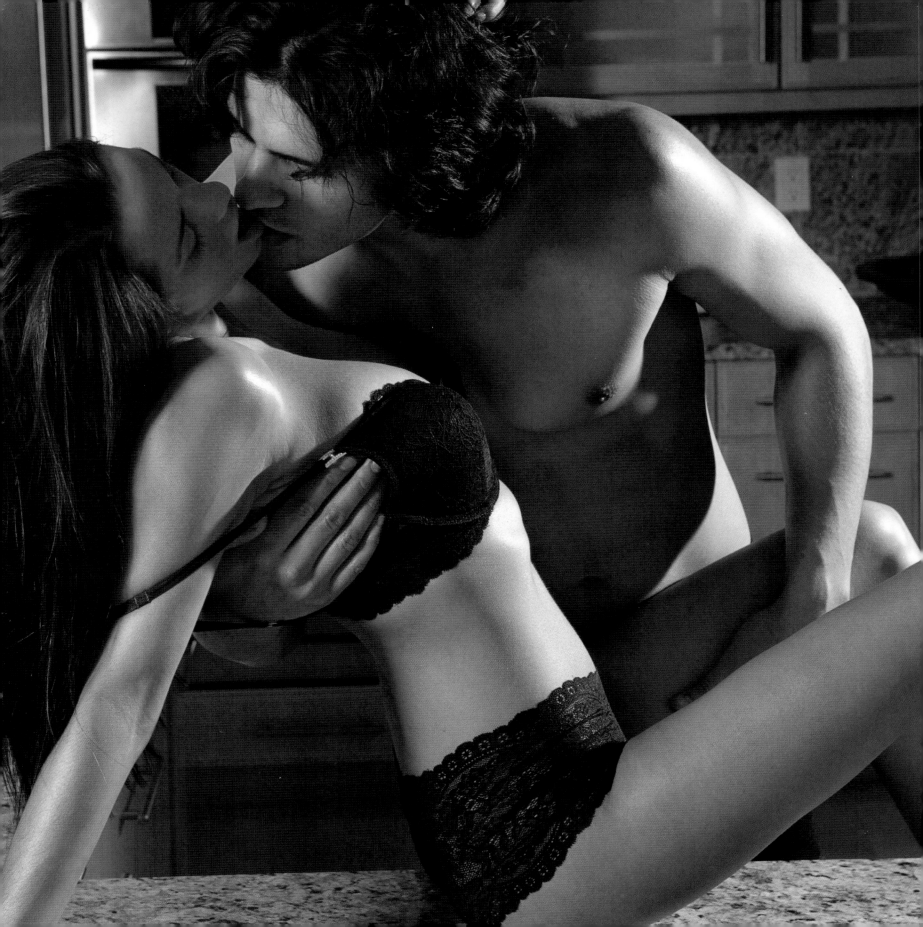

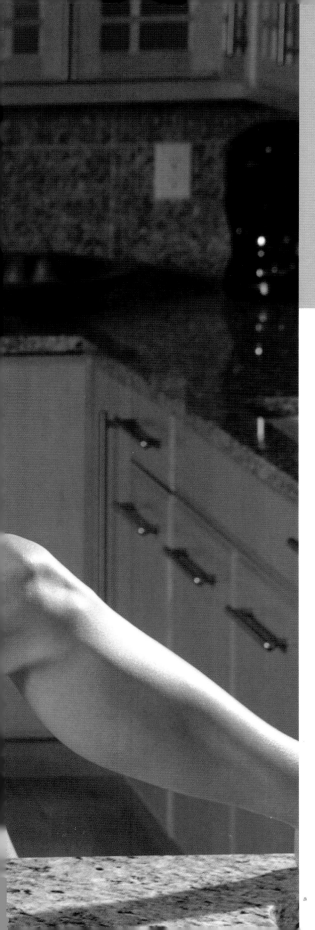

" Real talk "

"If you don't make a woman feel sexy, why should she want to have sex with you?" asks Anthony. "I find what is beautiful about a woman and focus on that with my eyes, my touch, my words, until she feels her own beauty. No woman feels sexy without feeling beautiful first.

"If I am drawn to her face, I let my eyes caress her features, run one finger down her cheek, cup her chin, hold her face in my hands, and massage her cheeks lightly with my thumbs. I praise her, but the words alone are not enough. It is the gaze and the tender touch that make her feel beautiful and desired—and sexy."

Generally openness to sexual possibility is expressed through an open body. But sometimes crossed arms are a sign of playfulness. Or the room is cold and the arms are bare. Maybe she's accentuating her breasts. Maybe he feels more comfortable with one leg crossed over the other. Don't read too much into one gesture that's been described as "closed."

Couples who have been together awhile also talk to each other through body language. Yet sometimes one misses the other's signals. Pay attention to your partner's unspoken cues and you'll make more of the right moves, and fewer of the wrong ones.

Some sex techniques are absolutely essential skills. You can't be a good lover if you haven't mastered them. The first of these essential skills is described in the box below. Pay special attention to these Essential Skills boxes. If you are adept at the essential skills, you will satisfy your partner and yourself. You'll be a good lover.

Everything else is hot-fudge sauce on the vanilla-bean ice cream. (Master all the techniques and you will be a *great* lover—an admirable goal.)

Shedding Inhibitions

Maybe you're a successful flirt but you have some problems with the follow-through. Something seems to be holding you back. Many people have sexual hang-ups to one degree or another. A seduction is an erotic invitation issued by a man or a woman who convincingly extends the promise of good sex to a partner. That's a difficult invitation to put out there if you are inhibited about your body or have performance issues.

If you're thinking, "He'll look at my fat thighs and get turned off" or "I won't be able to give her an orgasm and I'll disappoint her," you need to get inside your head and make some quick adjustments to the mental messages you are sending yourself before this seduction is derailed.

MENTAL IMAGING

Imagine your hand on his bare chest when he strokes your palm. Can you almost hear the intake of his breath in the pleasure of your touch? Picture her head thrown back in ecstasy as you kiss her wrist. Whenever you feel that nervous knot developing in the pit of your stomach and fears are running like mice in your mind, stop the thoughts racing. Focus on a positive mental image of your partner in a state of desire or arousal.

Or imagine yourself as desirable and arousing. See yourself running hands smoothly and expertly down your lover's body. Picture the best parts of your body. Now do you see your partner admiring them in the next shot?

ACTIVE FANTASIZING

Turn those erotic still photos into a mini mental film as you're gazing into his eyes, kissing her lips. Just as fantasizing can revive flagging arousal during lovemaking, it can also keep the mood going when inhibitions intrude. Play out the seduction in your mind. Because it's your private screening room, you can check into and out of the story anytime you want.

"Real talk"

"Ironically, fantasy can make the reality better," says Carole. "I use fantasy when I need it, to get my head back in the right place. Then I drop it and concentrate on the real experience. The first time I performed fellatio on my lover, I was great at it, because I'd fantasized the act several times already."

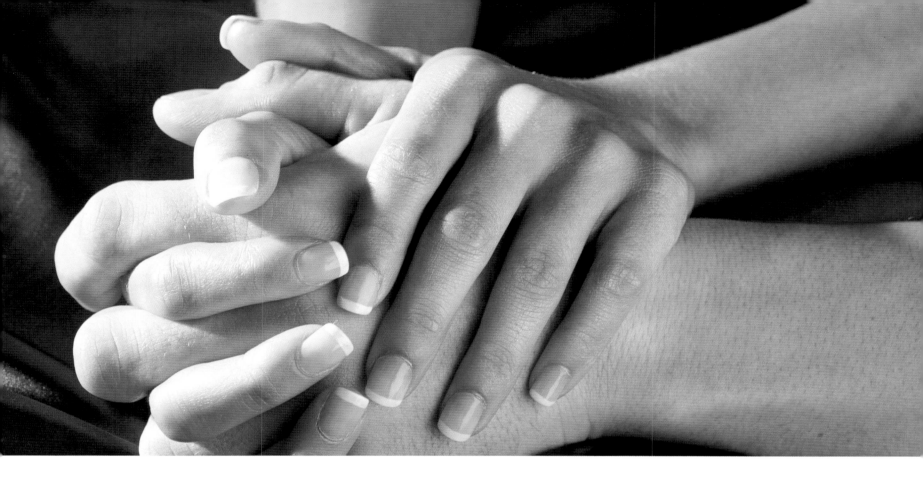

Creating a Romantic Ambience

THE BEDROOM

There is more to a romantic ambience than an attractive bedroom—but that space is certainly important. What you want in the lover's den are candles, flowers, clean and enticing linens, perhaps an erotic book, a lovely shawl draped over the foot of the bed, items that reflect your taste in art and literature. No dirty clothes on the floor, no dust bunnies in the corner, and no collections of dolls or teddy bears atop a dresser, armoire, or especially the bedside table.

THE MENTAL AMBIENCE

Your attitude toward romance, however, is an equally important part of the ambience. You have to be ready to have sex and let go afterward. Men lend themselves out to women—and take themselves back. Women too often give themselves away.

The prince and princess myths keep many women from being truly sexually empowered. They believe the prince will make them come. They think that having sex makes them an instant couple. There is still some truth in the old cliché, "She's pondering the possibility of a wedding while he's wondering how long is long enough for the postcoital cuddle."

But it is not true that women *can't* separate love and sex. Most women can. The secret lies in using the romantic fantasies when you need them—for desire, arousal, orgasm—and letting them go afterward just at the point where they would lead you to behave like a needy, clingy woman. Single women aren't the only ones who need to know how to separate love and sex. So do married women.

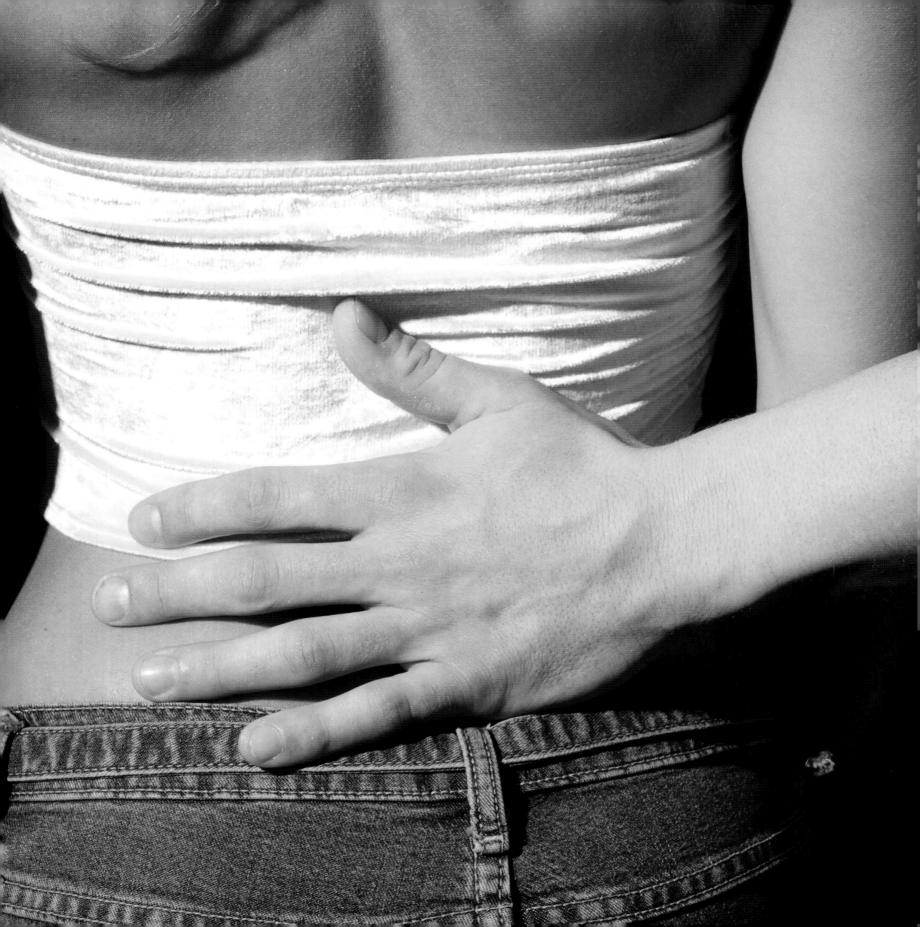

When a man places his hand on a woman's lower back, this nonsexual touch enables a woman to feel safe and comfortable, and allows the man to more easily advance to the next sexual level.

If you are angry with each other, he likely still wants to have sex. You don't. He sees sex as the way to make up. You see it as the reward for making up. This time he has the better idea.

Put your anger aside or transform it into passion. Try it his way.

Using Nonsexual Touch

Men instinctively know that touching a woman in a nonsexual way makes her more receptive to later sexual advances. That hand on her arm, shoulder, or back is a hand insinuating its way elsewhere. Psychologists call this "familiarizing touch." She becomes comfortable with his hands on her and accepts him when he presses further.

Women, on the other hand, are often expressing (or trying on) feelings of tenderness and affection when they stroke his hand or caress his arm. Her touch may be more playful than his. She is less likely to be concerned about whether or not the touch is welcome, because it usually is.

"Real talk"

"Think sexy," says Carole. "If you focus on your physical flaws or remember a bad time in bed, you wear those thoughts on your face. You project inexperience or unattractiveness—not the vibe you want to be sending. I know because I've done that, and it's death to seduction. He can *see* what you're thinking written on your face. A plain woman with a lot of self-confidence and a sexy mental attitude beats a beautiful woman with hang-ups any day."

STROKING

The lightest touch, stroking can be done with one finger or several. Use fingers or finger pads on the face and neck, back of the hand, lower arm, even thighs. Don't press too hard, and don't linger too long. A stroke is a tease, a promise—nothing heavy.

Tip: Stroking should be your initial touch. Concentrate on what you're doing. Feel the warmth and texture of the skin beneath your fingers as you glide over his or her body. You're not imagining it—your partner's skin is getting hotter.

KNEADING

A broader, bolder stroke, kneading in this context is not as probing as what happens to you during a massage. Knead shoulders, forearms, back. Slowly and gently squeeze the flesh between your fingers. Adjust your pressure to accommodate the amount of clothing your partner is wearing.

CARESSING

The most erotic touch—a caress—lingers on the skin. It doesn't run away like a stroke. Using fingers and the palm of your hand, caress hands, arms, shoulders, backs—and maybe chests and breasts if your partner is receptive and your space is private. Thumbs are important in caressing. While you gently squeeze your partner's flesh in your palm and fingers, stroke with the thumb.

" Real talk "

"If you are caressing a woman's breasts through her clothing and you don't feel and see a nipple erection, you need to back off," says Brian. "Go back to stroking in the safe body zones. Give her some space. Pay attention to her eyes. When they soften, try the caress again."

Technique Tip

Run your hand inside his suit jacket to massage his shoulders. That makes the act more intimate. If she's perched on a barstool next to you or has her legs extended on a chair or booth, firmly (but sensually!) massage her calves.

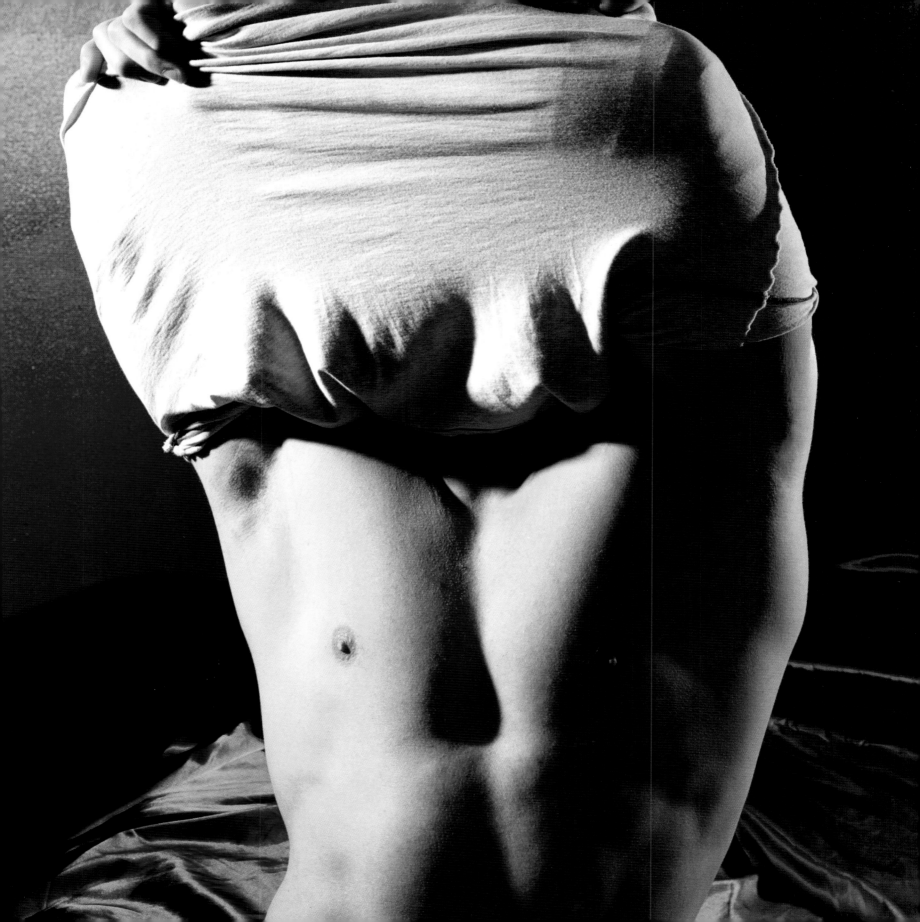

Sexy Talk

Not "dirty" talk, sexy talk is mental foreplay and includes paying more intimate compliments, making double entendres and suggestive statements, and asking very personal questions. You have to gauge your listener's comfort zone to know how far to go. There is a fine line between "sexy" and "dirty"—and everybody draws his (or her) own line.

And remember: Listening is also very seductive. Softly ask impertinent questions and pay close attention to the answers.

That works for couples, too. Get your partner to share a fragment of a dream or a fantasy. Or you do the sharing—and ask for a response.

A COUPLE'S STORY

Jeremy and Pam thought they knew everything about each other after eleven years of marriage. Then one night they were watching television together after their young twins were asleep. Flipping through a magazine, she teasingly suggested they take a sex quiz together.

"We were surprised to discover that each of us had fantasies we'd never shared with the other," Jeremy says.

"And I didn't realize how much he liked to perform oral sex," Pam says. "I thought he just did it for me."

That little magazine quiz led them to start talking more about sex. They asked each other questions and paid attention to the answers. Sometimes those answers were surprising—and exciting.

"It's a kind of preforeplay," she says. "Suddenly we realized that we had talked to each other this way when we were dating, but we'd stopped sometime shortly after marriage."

"Asking each other sexual questions led to more touching and kissing and definitely more sex," Jeremy says.

"The moral of our story," Pam says, "is never stop flirting and teasing and playing with each other, both verbally and physically."

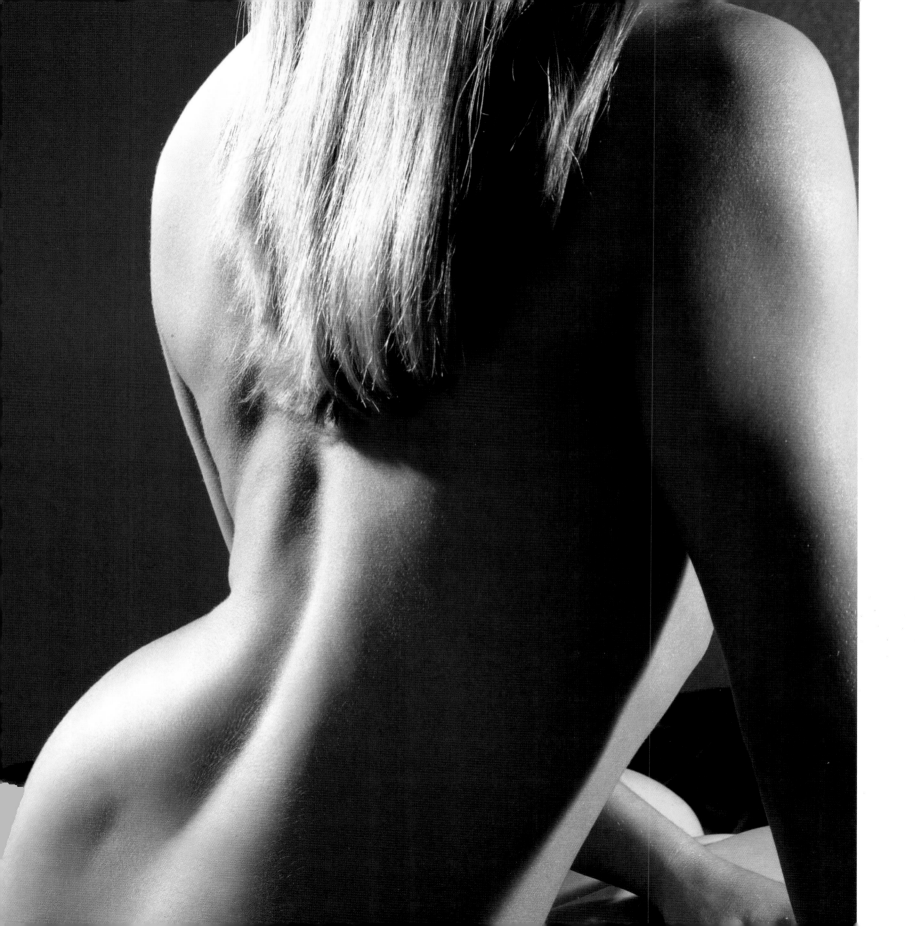

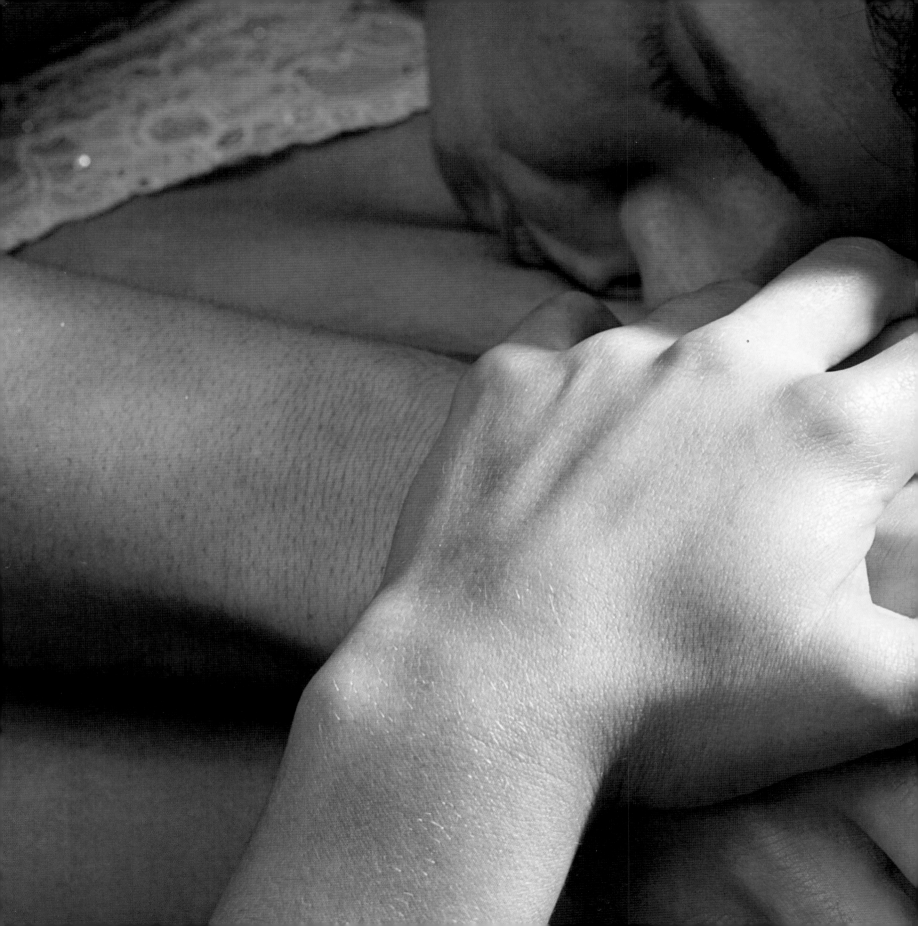

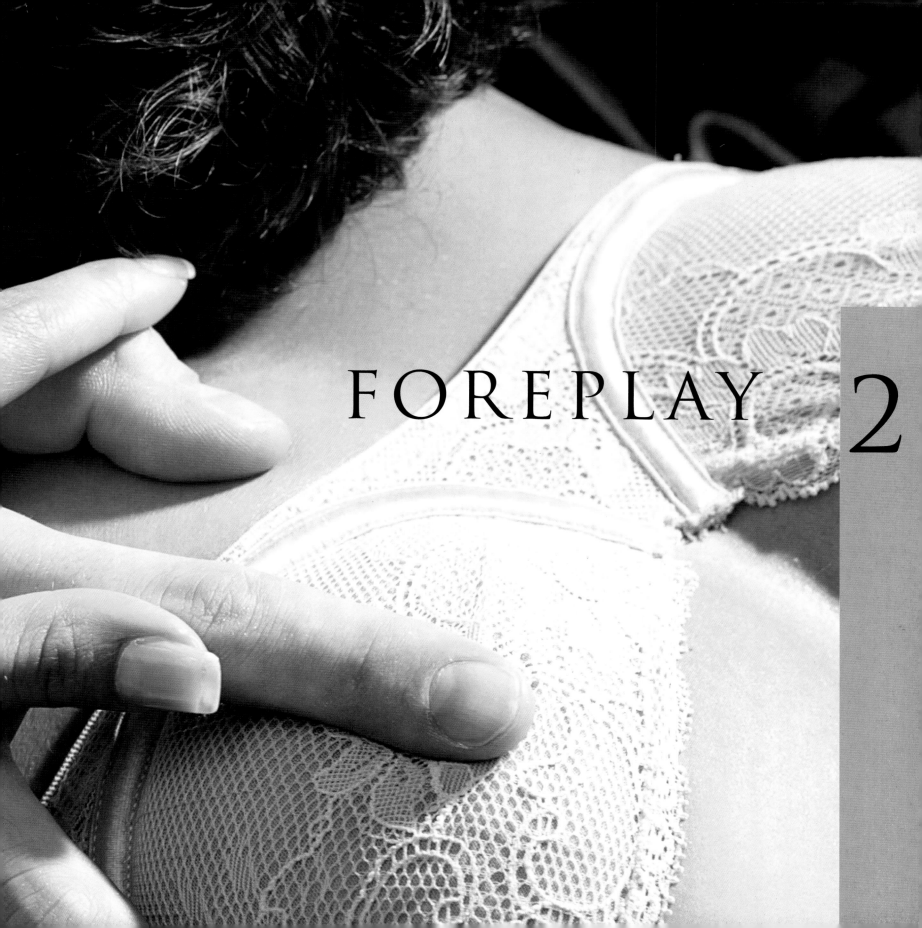

FOREPLAY 2

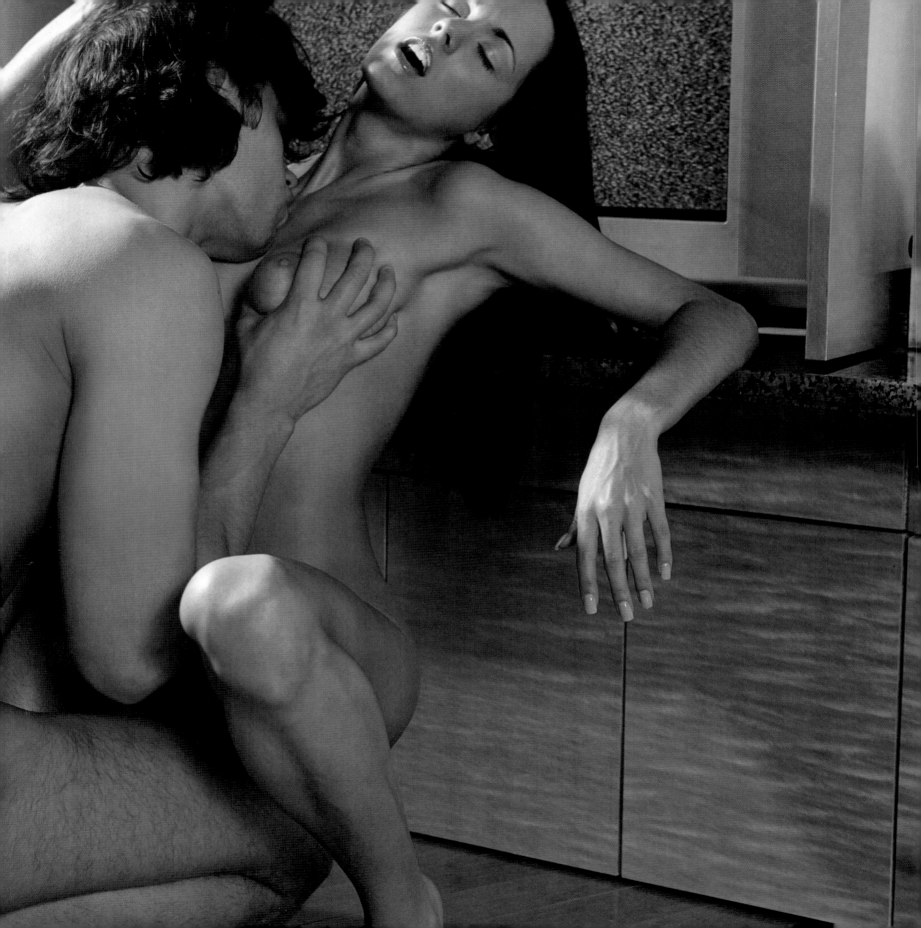

THE PLAY ONCE KNOWN
AS "FOREPLAY"

"Foreplay can turn good sex into great sex.

Good foreplay increases blood flow throughout the body,

heightening sensitivity. Every caress feels

more pleasurable when you're excited."

— Hilda Hutcherson, M.D.

MANY SEX THERAPISTS and other experts don't like the word *foreplay* because it implies that intercourse is the main or primary lovemaking event. They prefer *loveplay*, a term that gives equal weight to every erotic transaction and doesn't put all the emphasis on an erection. Whatever you call it—and most of us still use "foreplay"—that period of kissing, touching, caressing, and stroking is more intense and prolonged than the light and playful physical contact in flirting. It is meant to arouse—and more than a little.

We *need* foreplay to enjoy sex fully. That "we" includes men.

Glamour and *Men's Health* magazines ran the same reader sex poll in 2005. Not surprisingly, two-thirds of *Glamour* respondents said they wanted "more" and "better" foreplay. The *Men's Health* readers' response to the foreplay question may, however, surprise those women who still regard foreplay as something he does for her. Two-thirds of these men also said they wanted "more" and "better" foreplay. (More than a decade ago, when I surveyed one thousand men for the book "*Straight Talk from Men About Sex: What Men Really Want*," I got a similar response.)

It's time women got the message: Men love foreplay, too.

BEFORE YOU
(FORE)PLAY

Yes, there is something you need to do *before* the foreplay.

You will have better sex and more orgasms if you are in physical sexual shape to have them. The most important exercises men and women can do for their sex lives are Kegels. Often prescribed by doctors as the way for new mothers to regain vaginal tightness, Kegels develop the pubococcygeus (PC) muscle in both men and women.

There are also some exercises adapted from yoga that help women release the pent-up sexual energy in their pelvic areas—and a breathing technique to stimulate arousal.

None of these exercises are difficult or time-consuming—and they make a huge difference in your sexual performance and enjoyment. Kegels are an essential skill. You just can't get the most out of sex—or give it to your partner—if you don't practice Kegels.

The first two breathing techniques couldn't be easier to learn. They produce a lot of benefits for the effort put into learning and practicing them. And you have to breathe anyway, don't you?

Once you can easily perform the Breath of Fire, add Fire Breathing. Similar name, different technique. Fire Breathing can arouse you to a higher level than the Breath of Fire. And you will later need to know how to do this when I teach you the revolutionary Orgasm Loop. It's one component of that process.

The next two techniques target the pelvic area. The goal is to "loosen" the tightness in that region and infuse it with warm desire. Again, these are easy. Bonus: They feel good while you're doing them.

Technique Tip

FIRE BREATHING

Lie on your back, knees bent, feet spaced well apart. Start by taking deep breaths. Pull each breath into your body so deeply that you feel your diaphragm expanding.

Imagine this huge intake of air going all the way down into your genitals. When you exhale, push that air all the way out through your genitals and out of your body.

After a dozen or so deep breaths, pant by breathing rapidly from your belly with your mouth open. Do this ten or twenty times, then breathe deeply, inhaling through your nose and exhaling through your mouth. Make the breathing a continuous circular motion.

Imagine a circle of fire, beginning as a small circle composed at first of only nose and mouth, then expanding to include chest and belly in the next circle, and finally widening out to include the genitals. Feel the erotic heat moving throughout your body in a circle as you breathe. And feel your arousal growing with every breath.

Technique Tip

THE BREATH OF FIRE

The Breath of Fire is a simple way to oxygenate the blood, a process that increases sexual energy and elevates desire. You can use it before or during lovemaking to get you into the mood or increase arousal. It's particularly effective if you're having trouble getting aroused.

Take rapid, rhythmic, and shallow breaths through the nose. Keep your mouth closed. Breathe this way for one to three minutes every day—and, of course, during sex.

THE YOGA CAT

Get down on all fours. Inhale, becoming swaybacked, bringing your shoulders up and in, and lifting your head. Now exhale, arching your upper back and tucking the pelvis in and under. Draw your diaphragm up and in and pull your anal muscles up and in. Bring your chin down toward your chest. Repeat nine times. Rest. Do another set.

This next one borrows from yoga—but adds a rock 'n' roll component.

THE PELVIC ROCK

Wearing sexy panties and bra, stand in front of a full-length mirror, your arms hanging loosely at your sides. Breathe deeply through your mouth, all the way down to your belly. Imagine you are breathing air into your pelvis and your vagina—and breathing it back out again.

Start a forward-and-backward rocking movement in your pelvis. Keep your chest and back relaxed, not rigid. The rocking should remain centered in your pelvis. Thrust forward as you inhale, let your pelvis rock back on the exhale. Rock back and forth for three to four minutes until you feel sexy.

Finally, this is the one you really must do. No excuses. When you feel the difference it's going to make in your sex life, you won't want to make excuses, anyway.

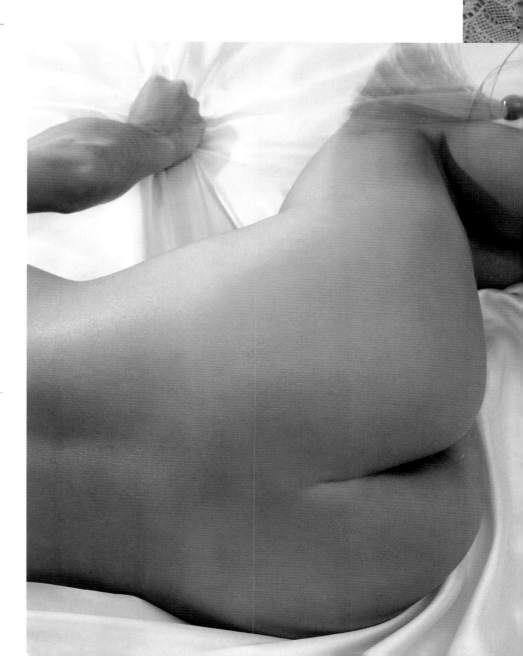

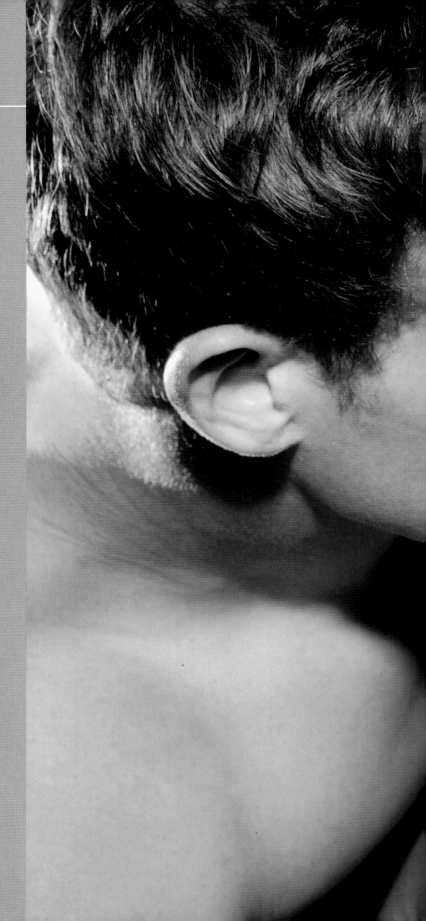

A COUPLE'S STORY

Like many women, Carolyn was disappointed in sex after childbirth. Her vagina was stretched. Intercourse didn't feel the same to her or to John, her husband. Her doctor recommended Kegel exercises. After a month of doing them, she found that her vagina was tighter—and more than tight, elastic, resilient. She felt sexier, more responsive, more in control of the erotic play.

"I could arouse myself to a higher level while he was kissing and touching me simply by doing Kegels," she said. "I had this new magic muscle. I'd learned how to play with it and I was having a great time."

John noticed the difference, too.

"Intercourse was better," he said. "And she was more interested in having it. She was hotter, sexier.
I would never have believed that doing simple exercises like that would make such a difference."

When she told him that men could do Kegels, too, he says, "That's all I needed to hear. I was ready to sign up for that program."

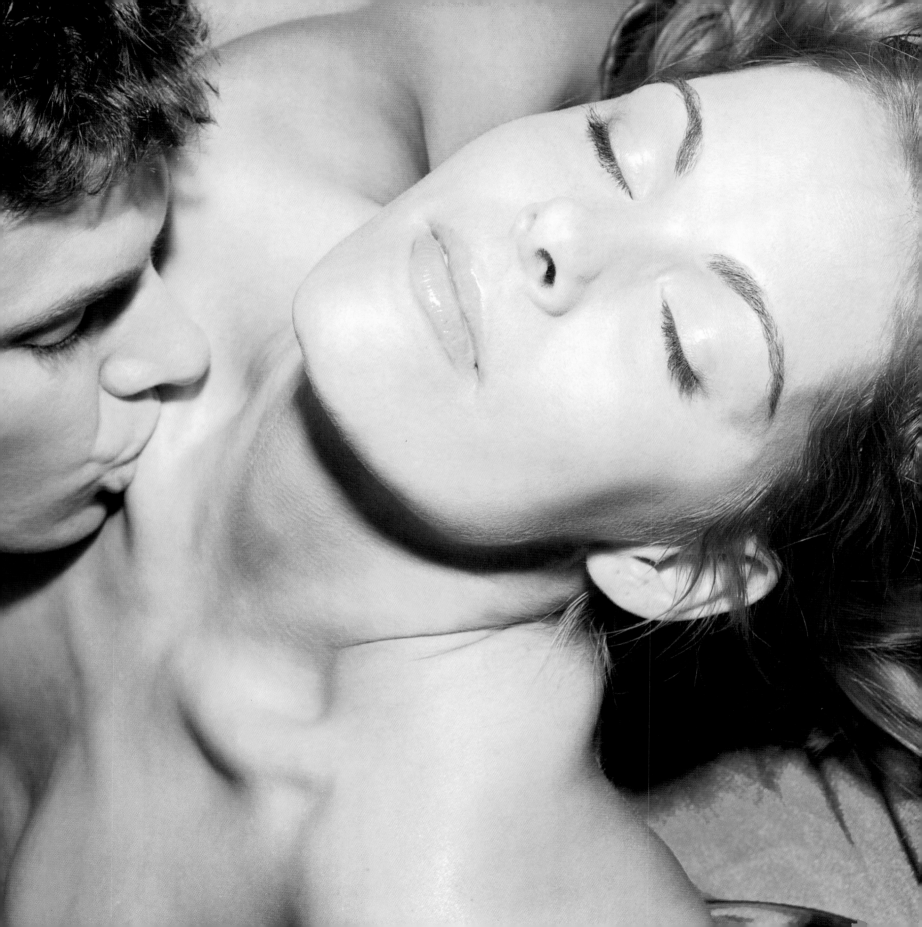

His and Her Kegels

Kegel exercises to strengthen the PC muscle are essential for men as well as women. Kegels are the absolute bottom line requirement for good sex.

Why?

- When you strengthen the PC muscle, you will have stronger, more intense orgasms—guaranteed.

- Women will have better control of his penis during intercourse.

- And can do some amazing tricks (see pages 94 and 144) by squeezing and relaxing her PC muscle around the shaft of his penis.

If you aren't already practicing these exercises, start now.

Then start with:

A SHORT KEGEL SEQUENCE

Contract the muscle twenty times at approximately one squeeze per second. Exhale gently as you tighten only the muscles around your genitals (which include the anus), not the muscles in your buttocks. Don't bear down when you release. Simply let go. Do two sets twice a day. Gradually build up to two sets of seventy-five per day.

Then add:

A LONG KEGEL SEQUENCE

Hold the muscle contraction for a count of three. Relax between contractions. Work up to holding for ten seconds, relaxing for ten seconds. Again start with two sets of twenty each and build up to seventy-five.

You will be doing three hundred repetitions a day of the combined short and long and be ready to add:

THE PUSHOUT

After relaxing the contraction, push down and out gently, as if you were having a bowel movement with your PC muscle. Repeat gently. No bearing down.

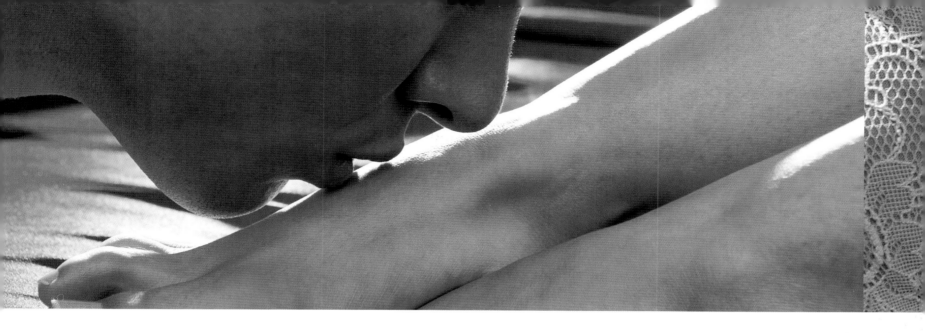

THE ELEMENTS OF FOREPLAY

Kissing, touching, stroking, and caressing are the elements of foreplay. Partners use their hands and mouths to stimulate and arouse each other. A cursory few minutes of deep kissing and groping genitals doesn't get that job done. Women typically say they would like twenty minutes of foreplay, while men want fifteen.

Kissing

Women's number-one complaint about the way men kiss: "Too much tongue."

Use the tip of your tongue. Outline her lips with it. Explore the tip and the edges of her tongue. Whatever you do, don't ram your tongue into her mouth.

Men's number-one complaint about the way women kiss: "Mouth not relaxed and open enough."

With lips parted and mouth relaxed, pay attention to his lips, one at a time. Lightly suck first his bottom lip, then the top. With the tip of your tongue, lick each lip. Now give him a full mouth kiss with relaxed, open lips and a little tongue. Hold his face in your hands and pull back slightly from him if he introduces too much tongue.

His favorite foreplay activity? Oral sex, both the giving and the receiving of it. Her choice? Kisses to her mouth, throat, neck, breasts.

THE FRENCH KISS

It's not inserting a whole tongue into her mouth. That is a tongue sandwich.

A French kiss *is* the most delicate interplay of the tips of your tongues. With the tip of your tongue, play with your partner's lips, tongue, inside of mouth. Lead with the tip. Pull back. Circle your lover's tongue with the tip of yours. Pull back. Repeat, repeat, repeat.

When you are both very aroused, thrust the tip of your tongue in and out in rhythmic, stabbing movement. Even when your lips are passionately locked, your tongues are not wrestling for control of the shared oral space. Only tease each other with the tips of your fast-moving tongues.

Technique Tip

Turn that hot kiss into a make-out session.

As you're kissing, don't let your hands be idle. Run them up and down each other's bodies. Let your caressing and stroking heat up as the kisses do.

Slide your hands up her shirt. Stroke her breasts. Unfasten her bra if you can do that easily.

Unbutton his top buttons and play with his chest hair as you're kissing him. Put your hand inside his shirt and caress his nipples with flat palms.

"Realtalk"

Calvin says, "My girlfriend was all about the mouth. She always wants me to kiss her during intercourse, kiss her during my orgasm and hers, kiss her afterward as I'm holding her. I thought she would not be excited by the wrist kiss, but I was wrong. She says it is the most passionate and tender thing I've ever done to her body."

The Seductive Kiss (That Women Can't Resist)

■ Cradle her face in your hands as you stand facing each other. Caress her tenderly with your eyes.
Go in for the kiss gently. As your kiss progresses, cradle her head and neck with your hands.

■ Lean her against a wall or a door. Take her hands and hold them over her head as you're exploring her lips, tongue, and mouth with the tip of your tongue and your own lips.

■ Nuzzle her. Bury your face in her neck, her cleavage.

■ Come back to the kiss. Take her face in your hands. Kiss her until you feel her melting into your body. Then just hold her. She'll take it from there.

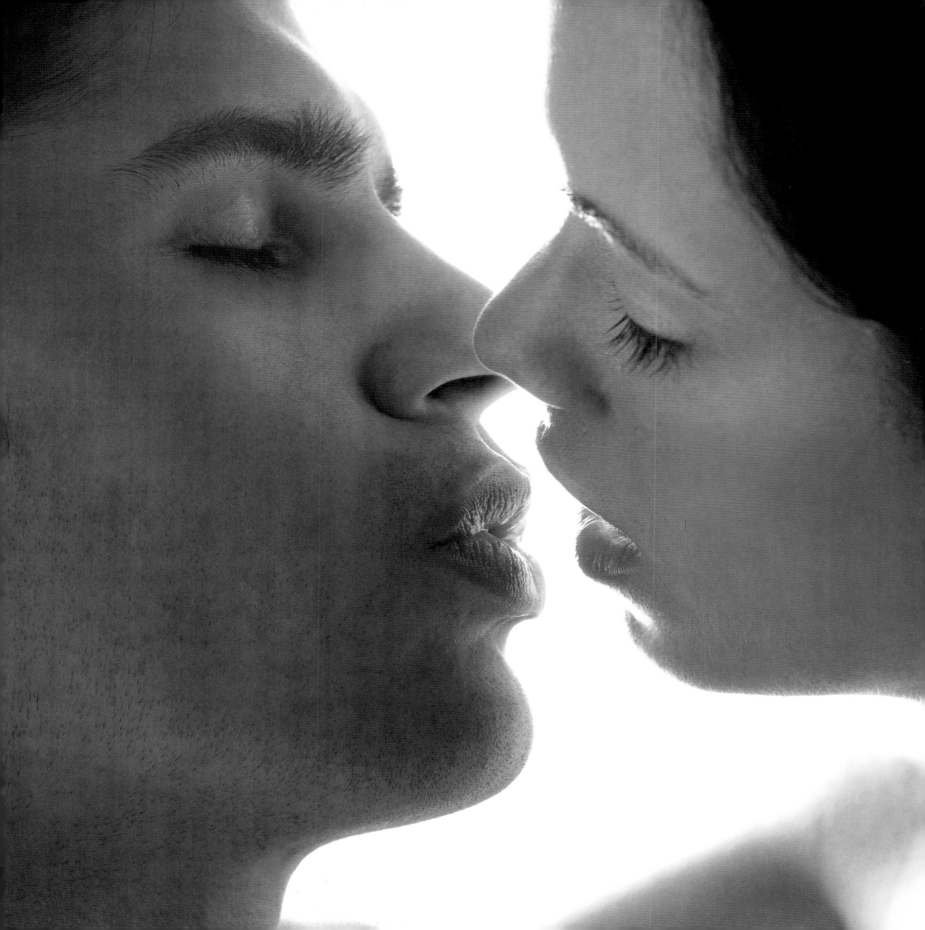

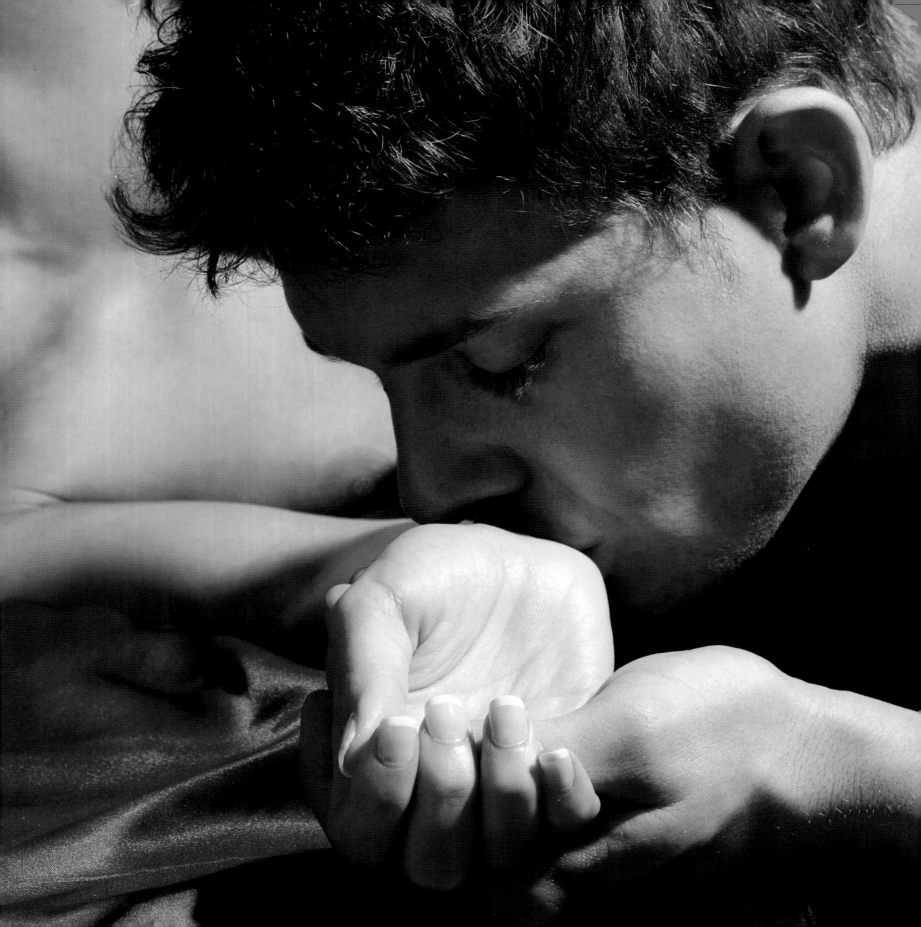

THE SEDUCTIVE WRIST KISS

Michel, the charming French gigolo who taught me this kiss, calls it "the ultimate kiss" because you can feel your lover's pulse on your lips. The instructions are written for a man kissing a woman's wrist. But a woman can kiss a man this way to great effect, too.

Kiss the inside of her wrist. Hold your lips against her wrist until you feel her pulse on them. Look into her eyes the whole time.

Brush your lips lightly across hers. Pull back. Take her face in your hands. While holding her eyes in yours, put your lips on hers and press gently, as you did against her wrist.

Close your eyes briefly. Put her wrist to your lips again and hold it there until you feel her heart beating wildly.

Now French kiss her.

"A kiss is sacred," says Michel.

"A man enters a woman's soul

through kissing her."

Eyes Open? or Closed?

Studies show that 90 percent of women close their eyes while kissing. Only a third of men do. Why don't women look?

We're missing an opportunity for more intense emotional intimacy when we keep those eyes tightly closed. And, by the way, shouldn't men get a little credit in the intimacy department, since they are trying to make eye contact while kissing? Men bond with a greater intensity if they can see into your eyes while making love to you.

You can also have a subtle influence on a man's kissing style if your eyes are open. He can see how his kisses are affecting you—or not. If not, he will naturally make some adjustments.

Combine eye contact with taking his face into your hands so you can gently pull him in or push him back. He's more likely to follow your lead if he can see your eyes.

Technique Tip

THE SCENT KISS

Perfume only the parts of your body you want your lover to touch. This may be the obvious places, such as the genitals, or those places you secretly wish she or he would touch more often, such as armpits, the backs of knees, inside the elbows. Have him or her sniff lightly to find the scent and then inhale deeply only those perfumed places. No touching. He is kissing you with his nose. Be sure he likes the scent before you do this. (Or she.) This is no time to try a new perfume.

Kissing Down the Body

If you have the time for luxurious lovemaking, kiss down your lover's body as you are undressing each other. Be sure you hit the "hot spots," those magic erotic places that are extremely sensitive to touch, oral and manual. You know where most of them are, but you might not be hitting them effectively, in foreplay, oral sex, and intercourse.

This is a good place for a hot-spot tutorial.

HER HOT SPOTS

- THE C-SPOT, her clitoris. The small pink organ, often compared to the penis because of its similar shape, is located at the point where the inner labia join at the top of the vaginal opening. The clitoris and the surrounding tissue, or clitoral hood, is the most sexually sensitive part of a woman's body.

- THE G-SPOT. That small mass of rough tissue about a third of the way up the front vaginal wall was named after the German gynecologist Ernst Grafenberg, who "discovered" it in the 1940s. In fact, the authors of the Kama Sutra wrote about this area thousands of years ago. The G-spot swells when stimulated and, in some women, produces orgasm.

- THE AFE ZONE. The anterior fornix erotic zone is a small patch of skin closer to the cervix than the G-spot is. Stroking the AFE Zone makes any woman lubricate immediately.

- THE U-SPOT. We don't think of the urethra as a sexy place; but the tiny area of tissue above the opening (and right below the clitoris) is a pleasure point. This is a good spot for him to stimulate if her clitoris is too sensitive for immediate touch following orgasm.

- INDIVIDUAL HOT SPOTS. Some women have very sensitive breasts or nipples. Other potential hot spots include inner thighs, backs of the knees, hollow of the throat, back of the neck.

HIS HOT SPOTS

- THE H-SPOT. Who doesn't know that the head of his penis is his hottest spot? Don't neglect the corona, that thick ridge of skin separating the head from the shaft. It is exquisitely sensitive to touch. Running a finger or a tongue around it can drive a man wild.

- THE F-SPOT. The frenulum is that loose section of skin on the underside of the penis where the head meets the shaft. In most men, it is highly sensitive to touch.

- THE R AREA. The raphe is that visible line along the center of the scrotum, an area of the male anatomy too often overlooked during lovemaking. The skin of the scrotum is very sensitive, similar to a woman's labia.

- THE P ZONE. The perineum is an area an inch or so in size, between the anus and the base of the scrotum. Rich in nerve endings, the perineum is the second most important hot spot for some men—and the most sadly neglected by women.

- THE G-SPOT. Yes, he has one, too—located inside his body behind the perineum. You can reach it in two ways: indirectly, by pressing the perineum with your thumb or finger; and directly, by inserting a finger into his anus and using the same "come hither" stroke that he uses on your G-spot.

Individual hot spots. Some men are very sensitive to touch in their earlobes, neck, inner thighs, temples, eyelids, nipples, and buttocks.

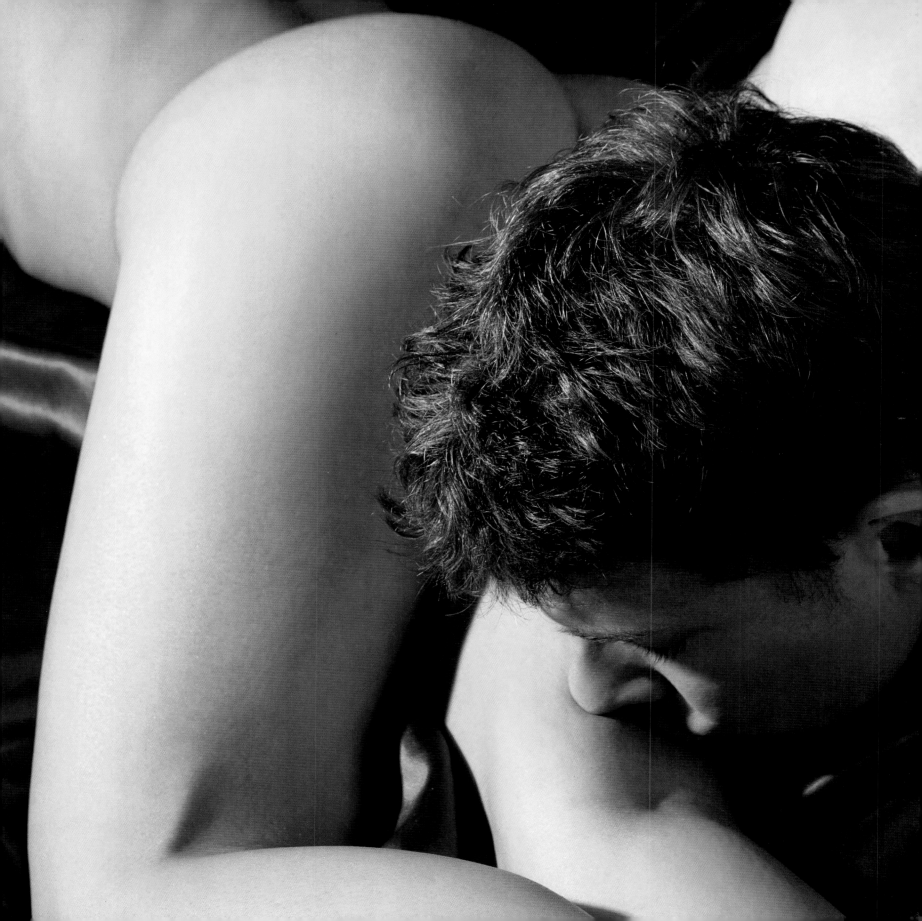

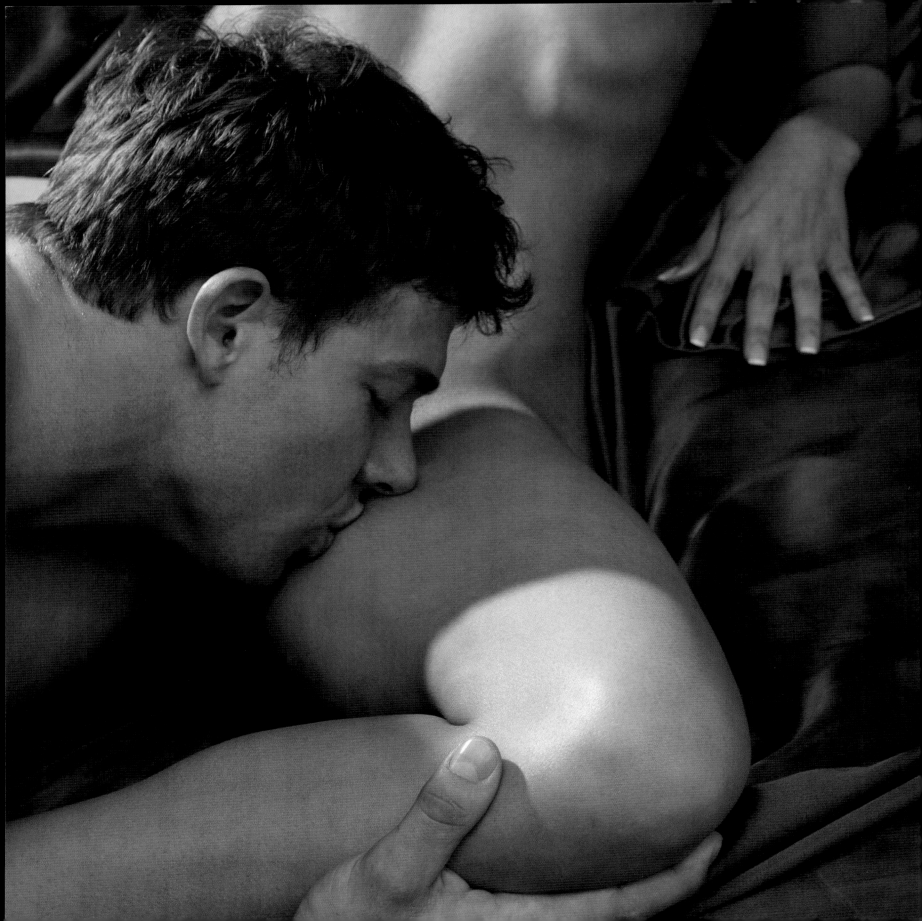

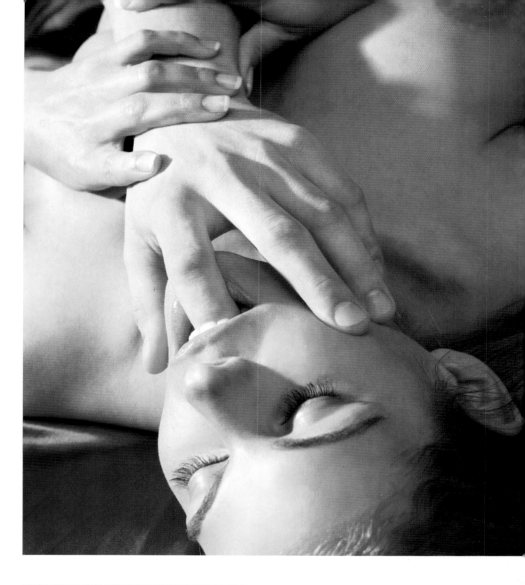

Employ both fingers and tongue to explore and stimulate your lover's hot spots. Pay careful attention to his or her responses. Use light pressure unless he or she indicates that more is desired. Expert attention to the hot spots during foreplay can lead to explosive orgasms a little later.

Combine the stimulation of hot spots by, for example, squeezing his buttocks as you flick your tongue across his frenulum—or play with her nipples while you are licking her inner thighs.

Sucking Fingers and Toes

Having their fingers or toes sucked excites many people. And doing the sucking excites others.

During passionate foreplay, take his hand, insert a finger into your mouth, and suck it in and out as he watches. Be sure your mouth is moist.

Technique Tip

This is also a sexy move to perform fully clothed in a public place. Suddenly the world recedes into the background. There are only the two of you and the promise of intercourse.

Kiss all the way down her body to her toes. Take each one into your mouth and suck gently for a few seconds. Stroke and massage her feet and legs as you do.

" Real talk"

Rachel says, "My husband used edible body paints to draw circles around my hot spots and squiggly lines down my inner thighs. We wrote numbers by the spots in the same paint. And I called out to him sequences of numbers for his fingers and tongue to touch—until I lost track of that and surrendered to the sensations!"

A COUPLE'S STORY

Tracy and Dean, in their early thirties, have been together for six years. Oral sex plays a significant role in their relationship. It always has. Yet in spite of their sophistication and intimate knowledge of each other's bodies, they only recently discovered hot spots.

"Like a lot of couples in our age group, oral sex was the first way we had sex—and, of course, we didn't call it sex," Dean says.

Tracy adds, "Because my early experiences with the penis were so up close and personal, I thought I knew everything about it. I was typical of girls of my generation in that I would rather perform a blow job than have sex with a guy I didn't know all that well. Naturally, I thought I knew it all."

Yet these self-described sex experts were finding their lovemaking growing predictable. They were in a rut. It was not a bad rut, of course, because they had pleasure and orgasms there. But they wanted more.

Tracy read about hot spots.

"What a revelation," she says, laughing. "That article opened my eyes in more than one way. First, I realized that we were getting the big sex picture but not the nuances. We were missing the fine tuning, the higher levels, the wilder experiences. And, second, I knew that our sex life would always be about learning and evolving. That was exhilarating to me!"

Dean shared her joy.

"We had a sexual epiphany when we began playing with the hot spots," he says. "I couldn't believe how much more arousing fellatio was when she moved that little tongue from one spot to another and strummed me like crazy. We just suddenly 'got it' about making the connections between our hot spots. And she's right about the bigger lesson in that.

"We knew that we didn't know it all and wouldn't know it all, maybe ever, and that was a very good thing."

Touching

Foreplay doesn't always begin with the kiss. Maybe you put your hand on his thigh as you're sitting side by side on the sofa or in a restaurant booth. You give him a little massage with your thumb and fingertips, a combination of pressing, scratching, and tickling. Then you squeeze lightly, move your hand up his thigh, and repeat the minimassage. He is aroused and you haven't done anything but play with his thigh.

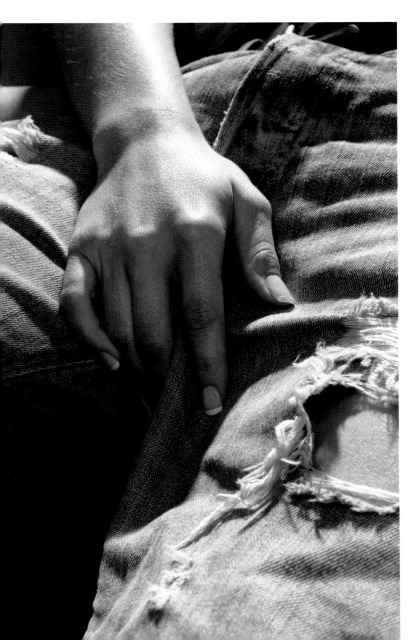

Good hands are crucial to good sex.

We use our hands to touch and stroke. What's the difference between the two? Touches are light. Fingertips dance and flirt across the skin of your lover. Meant to arouse initially, touches are less focused than the stroking that takes you to a higher level of arousal.

AROUSING HER SOFTLY

If you touch her the right way, you can probably change "not in the mood" or "too tired" to "yes." Don't start with an insistent touch. Make your approach to her soft and sensual. You might respond positively to her hand on your penis as an opening move, but she is more likely to get aroused by a more subtle approach.

If she rests her head on your shoulder, massage her scalp lightly with your knuckles or finger pads.

Stroke her forehead with the fingers of both hands from the center to the temples. Press lightly at her temples, then release.

Hold her hand. Caress the back of her hand with your thumb—the way you did when you were dating.

Hold her wrist, keeping your thumb on her pulse.

Now let her come to you, meeting your touches with her own.

"Good hands are crucial

to good sex."

ANCIENT CHINESE PLEASURE POINTS

According to ancient Chinese erotic texts, each of us, male and female, has certain "acupoints," spots that, when stimulated, boost sexual stamina and recharge sex drive. That may or may not be true for you. But touching the points will produce immediate pleasurable erotic sensations. It will make your lover be more sensitive to touch—and long for more.

Here are the pleasure points:

THE CINNABAR FIELD

A line of seven points from the navel to the front of the pubic bone, above the genitals. Imagine a line connecting the navel with this point—and containing five additional points, each equidistant from the others. Lightly press each point with a finger pad for three to five seconds.

NIPPLES

His and hers. Use your thumbs to press the nipples in—and rotate for three to five seconds.

BREASTS

Hers. Or his chest. On each breastbone, approximately nipple level, there are two points, on either side of and equidistant from the nipple. Use your finger pad to touch for three to five seconds.

GROIN

A pair of pleasure points are located somewhere along the crease between the abdomen and thighs. Lightly tap with your finger pads until your partner says, "Yes," and then press for three to five seconds.

THE MIDPOINT OF THE PERINEUM

Between the base of the scrotum and the anus in men and the vaginal opening and the anus in women. Press a thumb or finger pad against that spot and hold for three to five seconds.

USE YOUR FINGER PADS

The Spider's Legs is a highly arousing light touch, adapted from massage technique. Use the pads of your fingers as if they were spider's legs wandering up and down his (or her) body. The touch is light. It makes no demands.

In the Walk of Love, you walk your fingers around his body from one erogenous zone to another. Moving more slowly and applying a little more pressure than in Spider's Legs, you create highly charged electric pathways. Your lover hungers for more touch.

"Real talk"

"I love the way my husband touches me," says Karen. "When he puts his hands on me, I feel like I belong to him. I like that feeling. When he rubs his thumb against my hand at the movies, for example, I get wet. His touch calms me down, focuses me, arouses my sensuality."

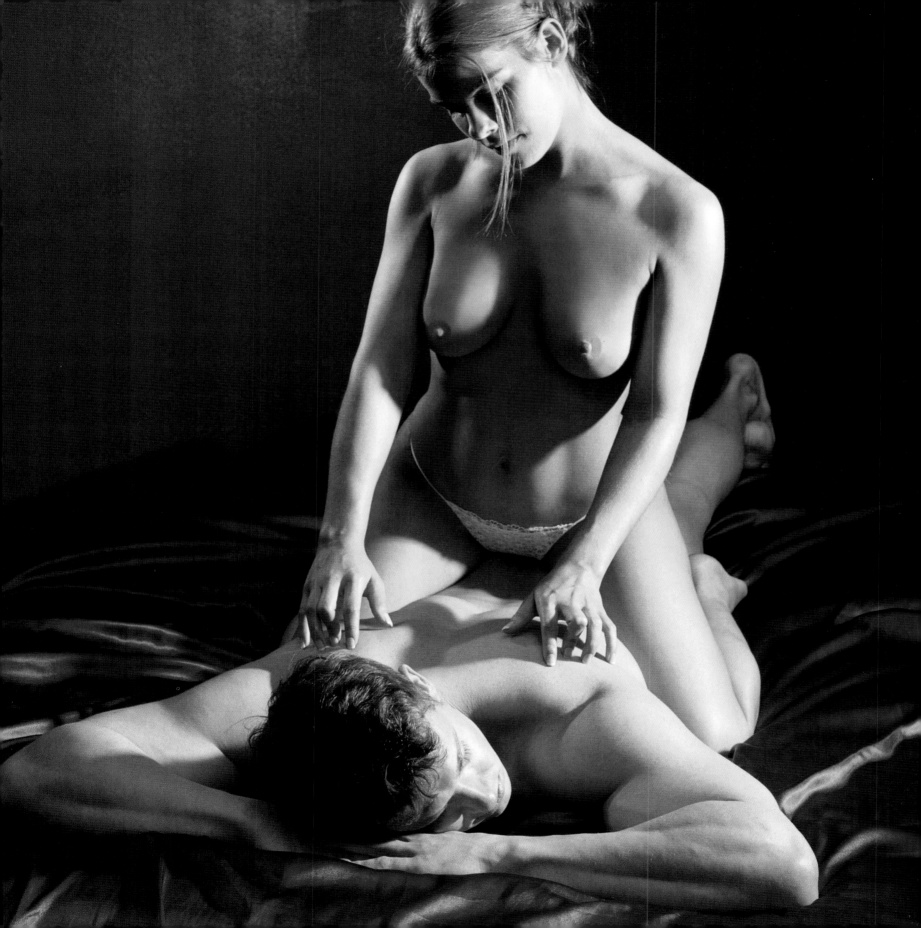

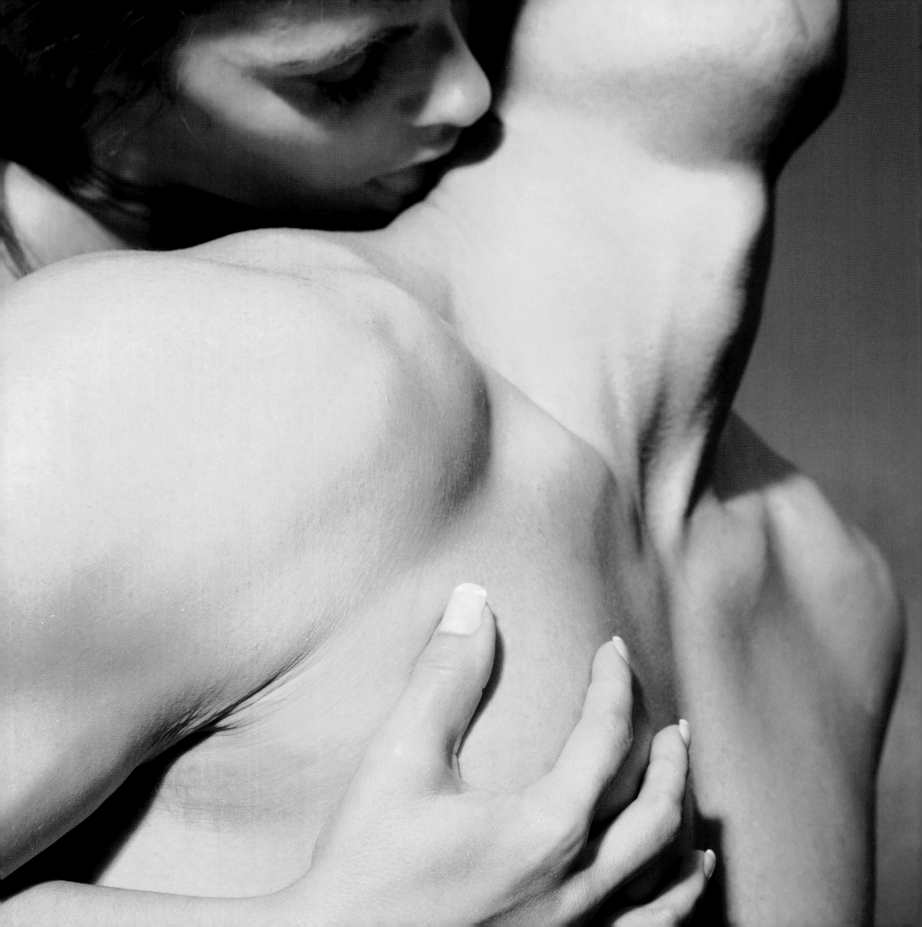

Stroking

The broad, flat strokes used in massage can also be adapted for erotic play. After touching lightly with finger pads, use the flat of your hand in longer, firmer motions. Those movements are strokes.

THE NIPPLE STROKE

Use the palm of your hand to brush lightly over her (or his) nipples. Gently rub her nipples between your fingers. Squeeze. Push them into her breasts, then gently pull them out, perhaps lightly twisting at the same time. Blow over her nipples with your saliva.

Now add oral play to her nipples and move your hands down her body. Kiss her nipples and areolae with light, flitting kisses. Follow by gentle nibbling. Run your tongue in circles around the areolae and nipples. Make the circles faster and faster. Suck her nipple into your mouth. Knead it gently between your lips, suck again, pull the areola into your mouth. Suck in more of her breast, as much as you can, and hold it firmly between your tongue and the roof of your mouth as you suck.

If you are a man who enjoys the same kind of nipple play, let her know. Guide her hands to your nipples. Cover her fingers with yours and show her how you like it done.

THE BREAST STROKE

There's an old joke about foreplay after marriage: Two squeezes to the left breast and a sloppy French kiss.

Stroke her breasts. Don't squeeze them. Massage them with the flat of your hand. Run your fingers up and down the sides of her breasts. Now run the flats of your hands up and down the sides. Caress them in both hands, push them together, and lavish attention on them.

"Starting in his thirties,

a man doesn't get an orgasm as soon

as she takes her clothes off.

She needs to touch him."

— Kim Cattrall, actress and
author of *Sexual Intelligence*

Adding the element of surprise is a great way to spice up foreplay. When a woman unexpectedly comes up behind a man, grabs his chest, and kisses his neck, there is no way he can resist her.

Caressing Genitals

The most common mistake women make in genital play is being too gentle. And the most common mistake men make? Not being gentle enough. We touch each other the way *we* like to be touched, not the way the other likes to be touched.

A warm-up caress for her involves delicate stroking of her inner and outer labia, perhaps allowing a finger or two to slide shyly inside her vagina while a thumb makes very wide circles around her clitoris. Imagine that you are softly coaxing her lubrication to the surface of her most private skin. You can't grasp her genitals and demand that they respond.

On the other hand, she probably can do that with you.

Take his penis firmly in hand. Stroke the shaft, caress the head. Luxuriate in the richness of that skin and let him sense that you do.

Initiate genital foreplay like a devotee at the altar of lust.

HOT SPOT FINGER AND MOUTH PLAY

Is she (or are you) frustrated because arousal is taking so long?

Insert one or two fingers into her vagina and stroke the AFE Zone until you feel her lubricating. Then massage her G-spot as you lick or suck her clitoris.

Now insert a finger into her anus if she finds that arousing.

For many women, the interplay of oral and manual stimulation, with special attention to the hot spots, is intensely arousing.

The Hand Job (such as he's never had before and couldn't possibly give himself)

- Clasp your lubricated hands together, fingers interlaced, snugly around the shaft of his penis. Move your hands up the shaft in one long twisting motion. Repeat the move back down the shaft. Now vary that move by eliminating the twist.

- When he has a firm erection, clasp your hands at the top of the shaft. Gently contract and release them around the shaft at approximately one-second intervals. Keep doing this up and down the shaft, stopping at the corona, the rim where the shaft meets the head.

- Alternate the twisting and contracting strokes until he is ready to ejaculate. Then hold him firmly in both hands, gently contracting them in time with his spasms.

- Finish him off by running your thumb from the base of the shaft on the underside up to the head.

A COUPLE'S STORY

When Emma and Matthew became lovers, they were, like many couples in their late twenties, "so hot for each other" that neither of them needed a lot of foreplay.

"In retrospect," Matthew says, "we were living in a state of continual mental foreplay for six months."

After they moved in together, they settled into a more typical pattern of lovemaking. Some of the urgency was gone, replaced by a growing emotional bond. But something else went missing, too: Emma's orgasms.

"We kept expecting everything to work the way it had before," she says. "He got an erection as soon as I took his penis in my hand. That was reassuring! Then we would kiss passionately, run our hands up and down each other's bodies, trying to generate the old heat, and caress genitals briefly before moving right to intercourse.

"When I didn't come, we thought he wasn't lasting long enough, but that wasn't really the part of the equation that needed adjustment."

They realized that they needed something they had used sparingly in the early days: foreplay.

"Never underestimate the importance of foreplay," Matthew says. "It's more than the pregame show—which is what guys secretly think. Good foreplay is what really gives a woman orgasms. Another big surprise: Foreplay doesn't have to lead to intercourse right away."

Sometimes they start foreplay in the morning—deep kissing, touching and caressing each other as they dress for work. Matthew calls that "priming the engines." Emma is more open and receptive to his advances in the evening because he has "put the idea of sex in her head and the promise of it later on her body."

And he spends ten to twenty minutes kissing and caressing her body and manually and orally stimulating her genitals. "I love teasing her clit with the tip of my tongue," he says. They don't move to intercourse until Emma has an aching desire for penetration.

"I make her beg for it," he says.

"And I do," she says—gratefully.

- Rub lubricant into your hands. Using a firm but not hard upward stroke with the palm of your hand, start caressing her inner thighs using your palms alone. Work your way toward her genitals with that same stroke. Gently part her lips with your fingers. Then stroke her inner labia.

- Be sure your thumb and forefinger are well lubricated. Use them to surround her clitoris. Massage. Some women like to have their clitoris stroked directly. If she does, take it between thumb and forefinger and gently rotate.

- Hold two fingers in the shape of a V and put them around her clitoris. Press down lightly. Pull back. Press down again and back up. This creates a rocking motion that may bring her to orgasm. If not, alternate the circular move around her clitoris, the rotating move (if she likes it), and the rocking V until she does reach orgasm.

Every good lover knows how to use his (or her) hands. The right touch is critical. Men generally want a firmer touch than women do. But let your partner be your guide.

Erotic Massage

When you have time for leisurely lovemaking, put all these touches, strokes, and caresses together in erotic massage. You may choose to take turns the same day or devote one session to her massage, another session to his. There is no better way for a couple to get back in sensual touch with each other.

One partner lies naked, facedown to begin. The other is minimally dressed, she in panties, he in briefs. Sparingly use lotion or oil that you warm in the palm of your hand before applying to your lover's body.

THE ULTIMATE EROTIC MASSAGE

- Begin with gliding strokes. Run your hands smoothly in long strokes that blend seamlessly together over large areas of his (or her) body. Don't stop to knead, rub, or fondle.

- Now make circular motions from the spine up and to the sides of the body.

- Knead gently—not with the vigor a masseuse might use—his shoulders and buttocks. Grasp the flesh into your fingers, then push it out. Don't pummel.

- Use single- or two-finger gliding strokes on his inner thighs, the back and sides of his neck, and, if he isn't too ticklish, under his arms.

- Have him turn over. Repeat the long, gliding strokes on his chest, stomach, and thighs. Use the single-finger stroke on his face, even the delicate areas such as eyelids and ears. Also run your finger down his neck.

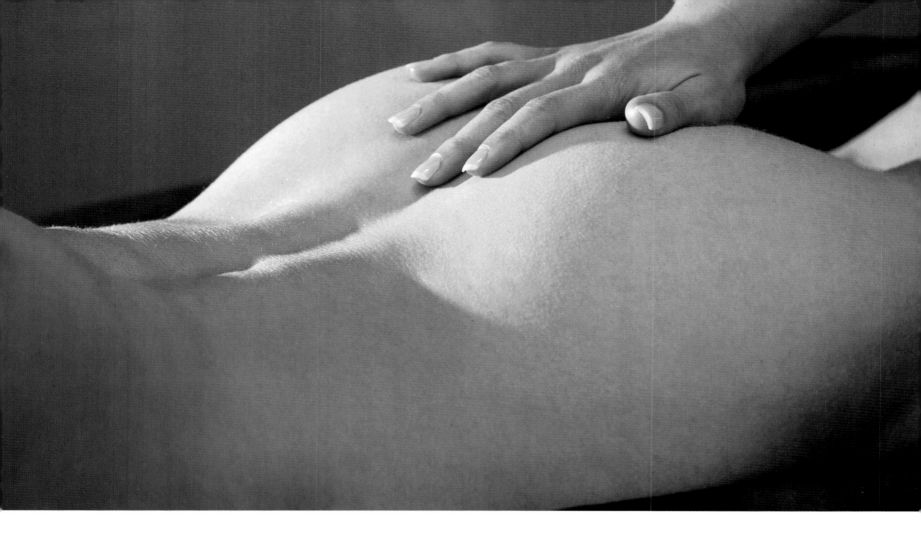

- Stroke his forehead with the fingers of both hands from the center to the temples. Press lightly on the temples.

- Now run your hands in broad, gliding strokes all the way down his body to his toes.

HIS GENITALS

- At this point, he probably has an erection. Straddle it, but don't insert it. Lower your breasts to his body and tease his nipples by rubbing yours across his. Or take your nipples in hand and rub them across his.

- In the straddle position, move down his body so that you end up kneeling between his legs. Gently take his testicles, one at a time, between your fingers and thumb. Then hold a testicle in the palm of your hand and tickle it lightly with the pads of your fingers. Now the other one.

- Hold the base of his penis in one hand and work your other hand in a circular fashion to the head. Use the palm of that hand to caress the head of his penis.

- As if you were building a fire with his penis as the stick, use a rolling/rubbing motion, starting at the base. Roll/rub up to the head and back down to the base, keeping his penis between your palms. Start slowly. Increase speed and pressure as he gets close to orgasm.

- Lean forward so that he ejaculates onto your breasts. To make him come quickly, insert a finger into his anus and press gently.

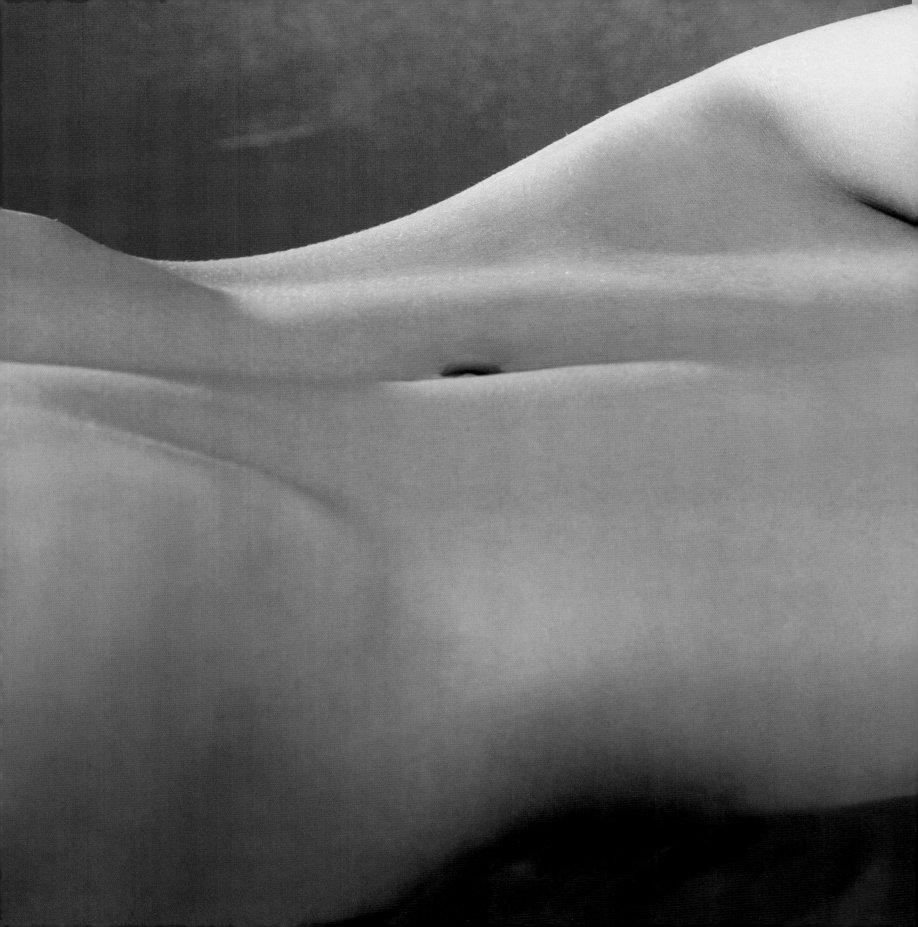

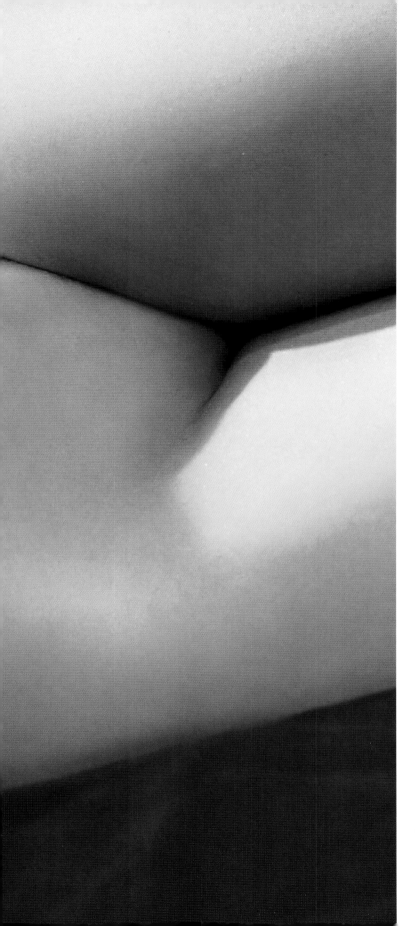

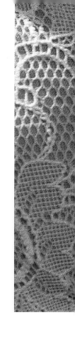

HER GENITALS

- Stroke her pubic hair if she hasn't shaved or waxed it off.

- Use light circular motions with your fingertips to make long strokes on the outside labia. Then curve one or two fingers and use the space between knuckle and joint to massage lightly her inner and outer lips in a back-and-forth motion. Massage her labia and work down to her anus.

- Alternate that stroke with one using your thumb or first finger alone.

- Rotate your fingers around her clitoris. Stroke down with one finger on either side of her clitoris. Rotate. Stroke down.

- If she likes that direct clitoral stimulation, you can take the clitoris between two fingers and gently rotate. But if, like many women, she can't stand the intensity of that stroke, circle your fingertips above the clitoris (at the twelve-o'clock point).

- Add the G-spot stroke. While continuing the twelve-o'clock rotation, insert a finger or two into her vagina and then massage her G-spot by making the "come hither" tickling motion toward her belly button.

- Now circle your fingertip rapidly around her clitoris as you're massaging her G-spot. Don't be surprised if she ejaculates with this orgasm.

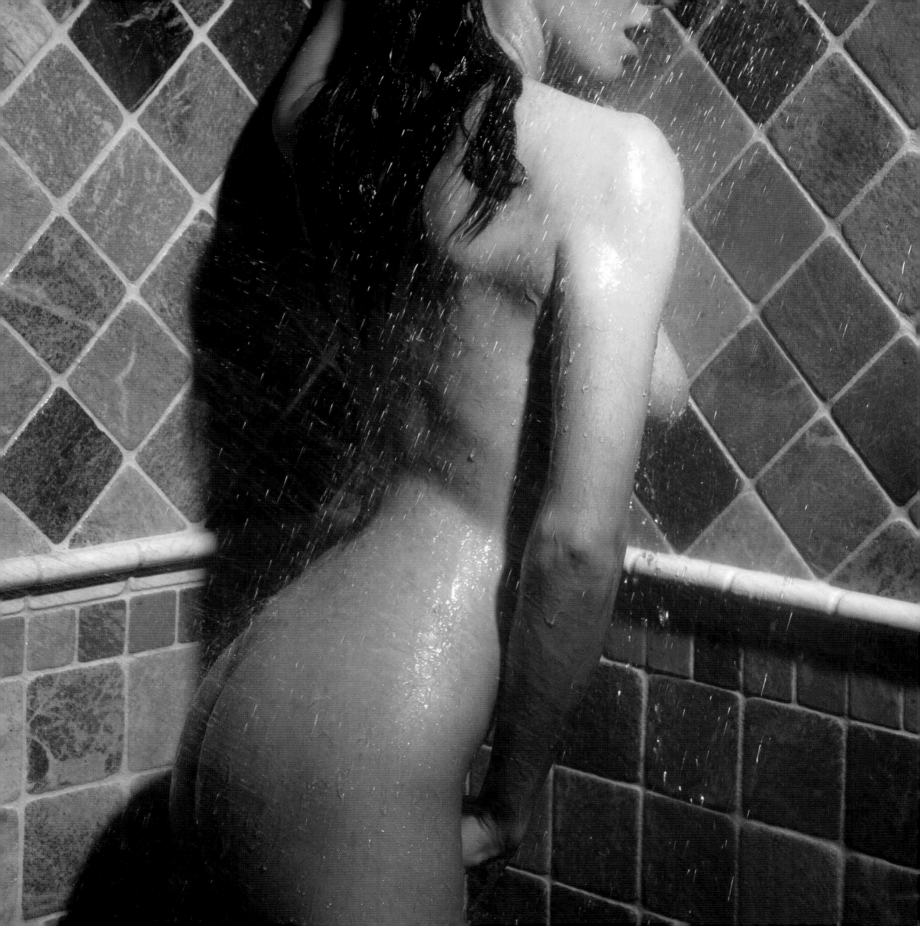

Games Couples Play

Sometimes you can really turn each other on by playing the way you did when you were young, before "sex" was a given.

Women love to make out. All that kissing, touching, stroking, and caressing before intercourse makes it more likely they will reach orgasm. But men love it, too. After the age of thirty-five, they need more foreplay to become aroused, especially in long-term relationships. Making out is pure play. Most adults need to play more often than they do.

These games will make you feel like kids again.

BUMP AND GRIND

Standing fully dressed, kiss and caress each other with your pelvises pressed together. When you feel the steam rising between the two of you, she bumps into him on the upstroke and grinds into him on the downstroke. Wrap one leg around his waist or use a door or a wall for balance. But don't lie down.

OUTERCOURSE

Do this on the floor, the sofa, or even in the bathroom. You can remove or unbutton shirts, but the pants stay on. Tease and stroke each other's genitals through the clothes. Lick, kiss, nibble above the waist. Get into an intercourse position, either one on top, and simulate the action. Move fast and hard. See if you can stop before you reach orgasm.

MUTUAL MASTURBATION

Watching her masturbate is probably high on his sexual wish list. Maybe it's not so high on hers, but she may be surprised at how much it does excite her. The bonus: Each may learn something about the other's arousal process. And she may feel more comfortable touching herself during intercourse when she needs that boost to orgasm.

Some women have never seen a man ejaculate in real life, only in porn films. Ejaculating for her is a very intimate act. And many women find it arousing not only physically but mentally and emotionally.

Ask her if it's okay to rub the ejaculate into her breasts. If she likes that, she may want you to ejaculate onto her breasts, stomach, or thighs—even her face. Just remember to keep it out of her eyes.

As a variation, masturbate, each of you with eyes closed, lying side by side so close you can touch (but you don't). Let your senses—smell, sound—excite your imagination about what your lover is doing. Or take turns masturbating while being kissed, held, and caressed by your lover.

"I love watching my wife masturbate," says Rob. "She has this little dramatic flourish when she's close to the finish line . . . swirling her fingers in bigger, hotter circles. I can feel the steam coming off her."

"Real talk"

"Mutual masturbation is a very intimate act," says Kate. "I thought it would be cold and clinical with each of us watching the other like a voyeur. It's not like that at all. There is something very special about opening yourself up to your lover in this way. This is sharing the most secret part of you, more intimate in a way than making love. I was very aroused and also very moved."

Throw yourself into masturbation with abandon. If you have the kind of headboard that permits it, put one hand over your head and grasp a rung or bedpost. Thrust your pelvis forward. Pant and moan.

Add some flashy moves such as:

- The Figure Eight. Use one finger to glide up, over, and around your clitoris, as if you were tracing the number eight.

- The Two-Finger Thrill. Hold two fingers parallel on ether side of your clitoris. Run them up and down and then sideways.

And don't be shy about incorporating a vibrator into your solo performance. It's a reliable way of reaching orgasm. And, by watching, he may get some ideas on how to use the vibrator to pleasure you.

Mental Foreplay

The mind is the primary sex organ. In men, the mind–body connection may be more direct and simple than it is in women. He becomes aroused by visual stimulation, for example, while she typically needs some words to go with the pictures. But both men and women have to be mentally aroused to make sex work. Don't neglect the mind in foreplay.

All foreplay activities have a mental component, some more than others. Teasing is meant to put the idea of sex into your lover's mind as well as get her juices flowing (or his erection throbbing). To paraphrase a sentiment made famous by one of our presidents: A mind is a terrible thing to waste in foreplay.

FLAUNT YOUR STUFF

Men want to be voyeurs. We instinctively know that when we're dating them. When we live with them, we forget. While talking to him (about anything), smooth lotion onto your bare arms or legs. Or lift your hair off your neck as though you're trying to let some of your sultry body heat escape. Or adjust your bra strap.

Old tricks—but they work every time.

TEASING

Like flirting, teasing as a part of foreplay is a lost art within "the relationship." When men and women are new to each other, they tease naturally by offering the promise of erotic delights, seemingly pulling the offer back, then slowly and suggestively putting it out there again. Teasing makes a woman feel naughty and dangerous and definitely in erotic control. And it gives men a chance to yearn for contact.

THE SLOW STRIP

The key is to keep your eyes locked onto your partner while removing your clothes. Wear clothes that can be removed to good visual advantage. No dresses that come off over your head, for example, or tight pants. Blouses and shirts that can be unbuttoned to reveal sexy lingerie—another cliché that always works.

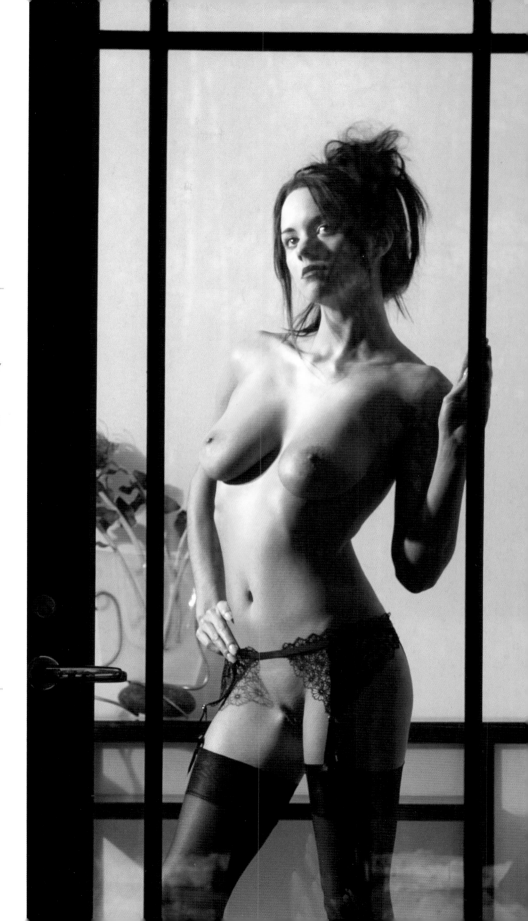

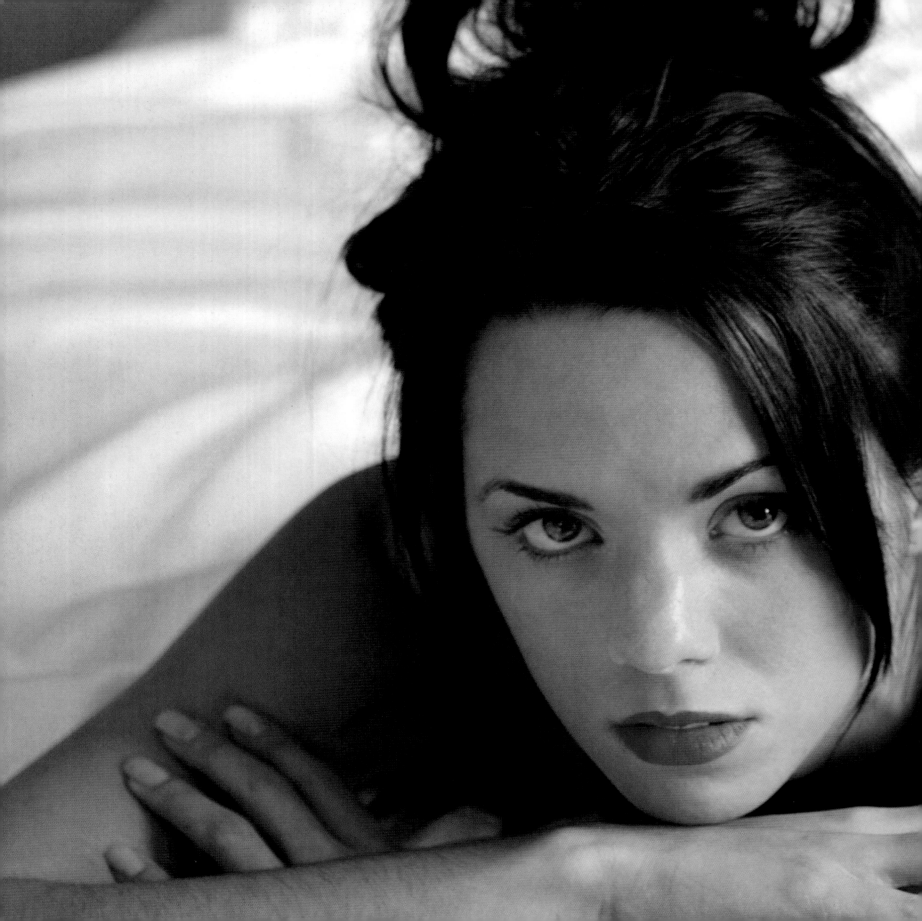

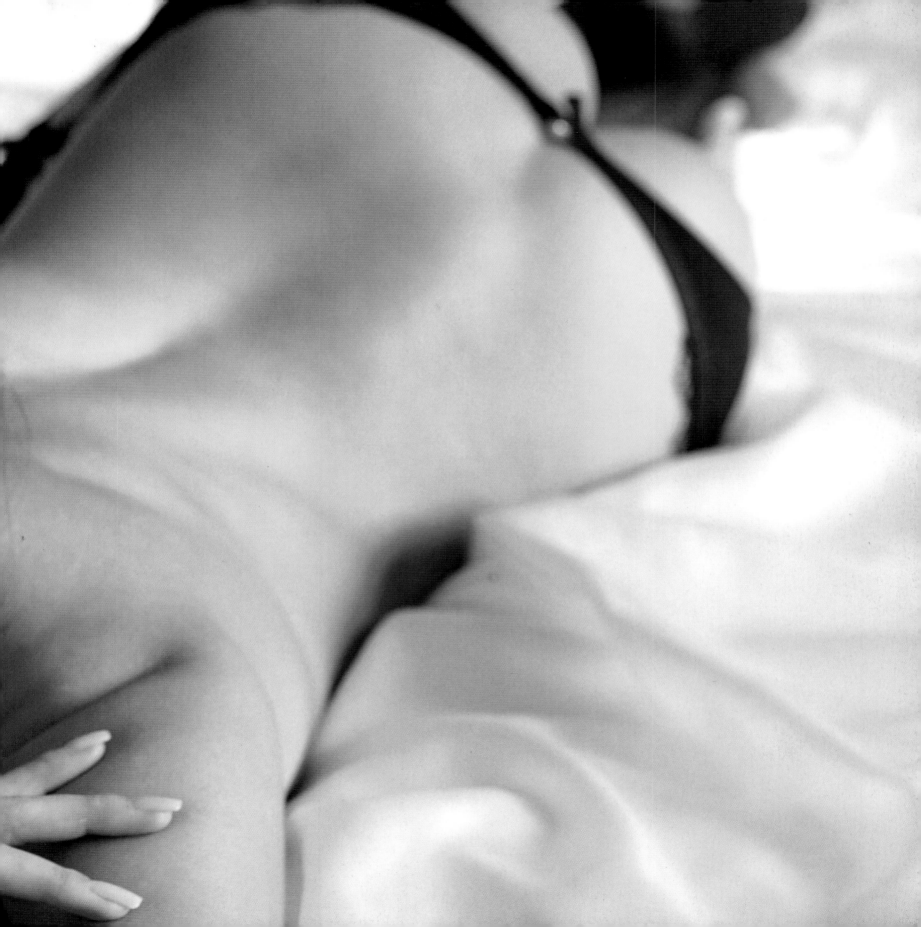

While the visual tease is most effectively used by a woman, both genders can physically tease each other. Again, remember how you played in the early days. Put the play back into sex play.

For example, take a calligraphy pen or a feather and tease your naked partner, paying particular attention to the genitals. Keep an array of sensual objects in the nightstand drawer. Buy a feathered mask and wear it while performing oral sex. The feathers dance and tickle in unexpected ways.

Or try perfuming only the parts of your body that you want your lover to touch. First, he or she must sniff, then touch.

Start the foreplay hours in advance. As you're heading out the door in the morning, lightly flick his nipples through his shirt or tap the head of his penis trapped inside his pants. Liven up the good-bye kiss by cupping her buttocks and pulling her passionately to your body. Whisper suggestive comments in his ear. Then go.

And, finally, add some love bites, pinches, and slaps to the foreplay when you get back together that night.

" Real talk"

"My girl knows how to turn my mind to sex," says Mark. "We can be in a public place and she'll take something off to get me going. She'll declare herself 'hot,' look into my eyes in that smoldering way, and remove her jacket, undo the top buttons of her blouse—with her eyes on me the whole time. As soon as the lights go down in a movie theater, she kicks off a shoe and runs her foot up my leg."

Technique Tip

An occasional bite, pinch, slap, squeeze—always done lightly, in the spirit of play—intensifies arousal for some men and women. Slaps are particularly effective on the buttocks, because they bring the blood closer to the surface of the skin, making the flesh more sensitive to the touch. But this is highly individualistic. Your partner may enjoy, for example, having nipples teased by love bites or pinches. Or she (or he) may hate it. Running a fingernail down the skin can also be very arousing (or annoying).

Pay close attention to your partner's reactions.

Foreplay doesn't necessarily always have to include masturbation, teasing, games, or erotic massage. Stimulation can occur from a couple simply sharing physical and emotional intimacy.

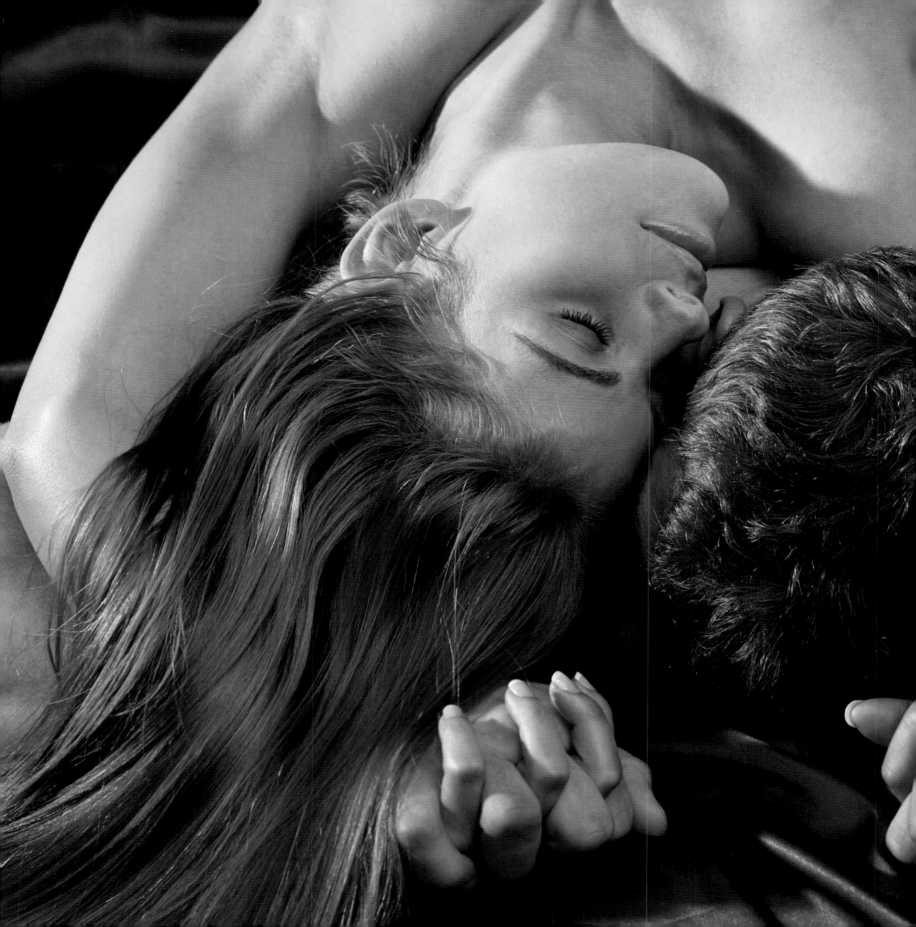

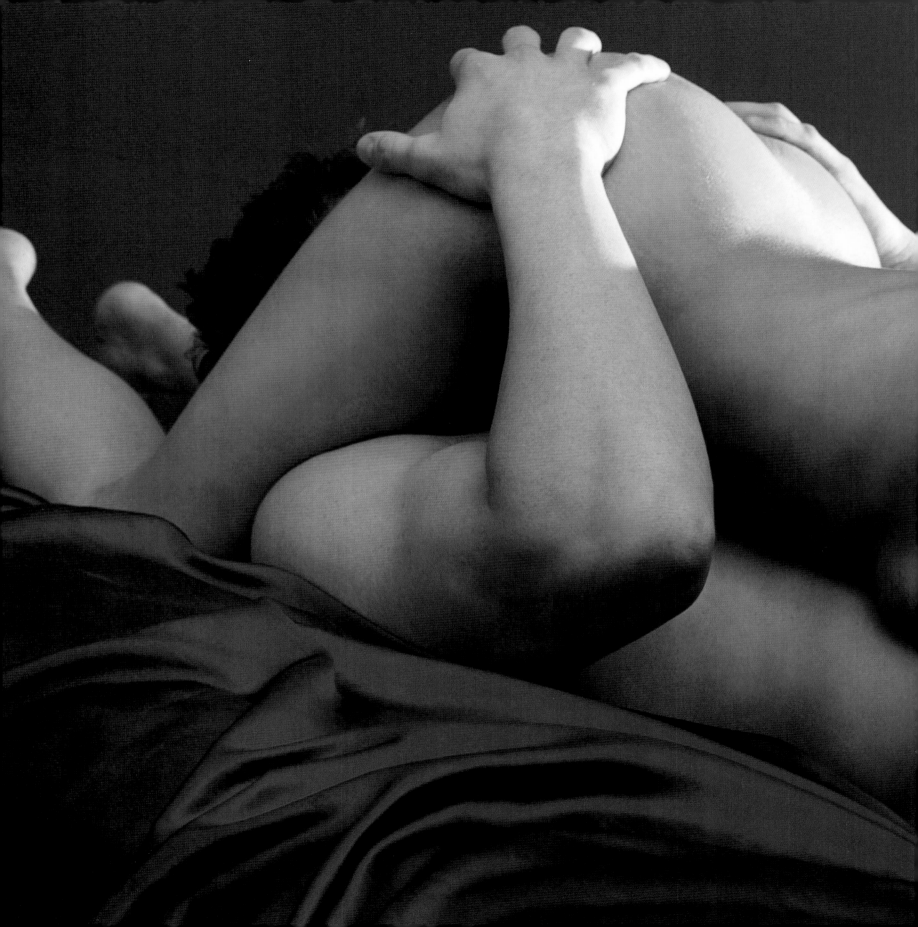

THE ORALS

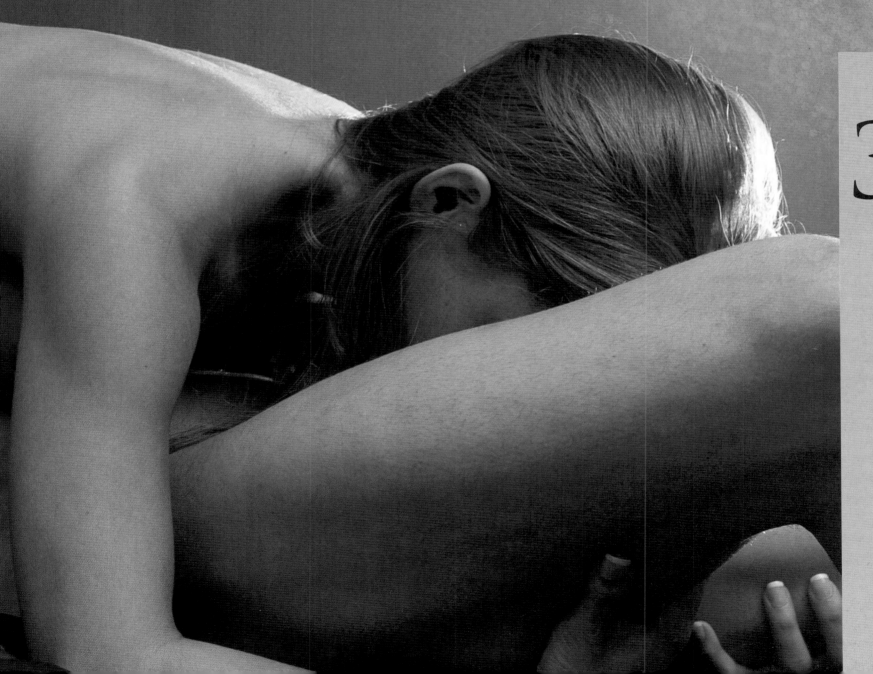

3

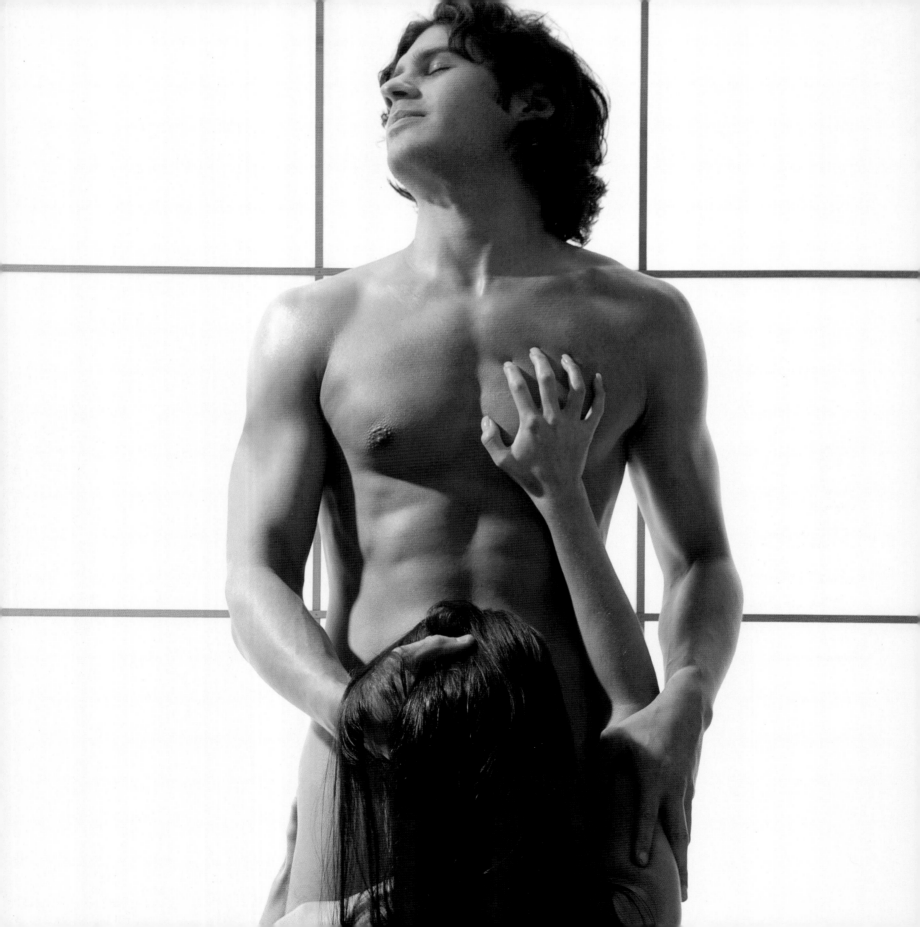

POWER OF THE ORALS

"Fellatio is the deal breaker.

It's not a sex life without fellatio."

— Jeff, a happily married man

ORAL SEX is foreplay if you stop before orgasm, especially *his* orgasm. Many men like to give their partners an orgasm via cunnilingus before intercourse. If she doesn't reach orgasm during intercourse, she has been satisfied before he takes his release. And if she does, she is in a good position for multiple orgasms.

When both partners reach orgasm via oral stimulation, oral sex quite often *is* the sex. There's nothing wrong with that. Intercourse need not be part of every sexual encounter.

Fellatio

Men love receiving oral sex. They are grateful for almost any efforts on your behalf. But every woman should know how to perform a blow job that leaves a man feeling extremely grateful. Even if you're not as into doing it as he is into having it done, you will thrill to your own erotic power once you see how this affects him.

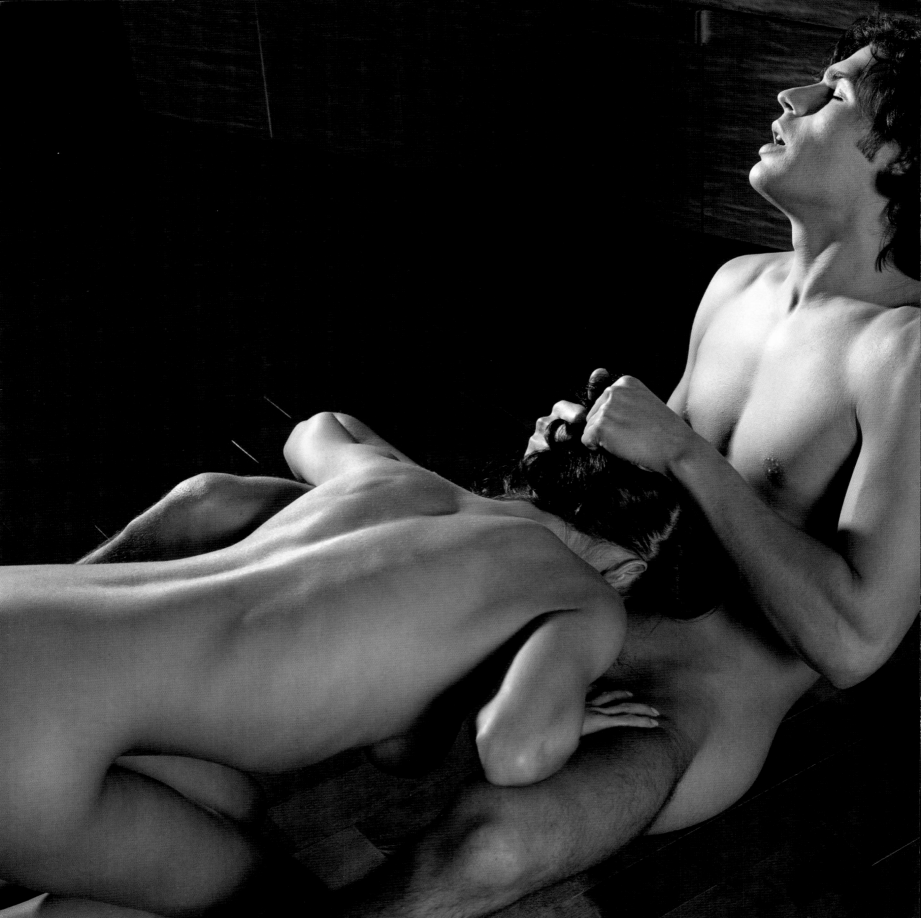

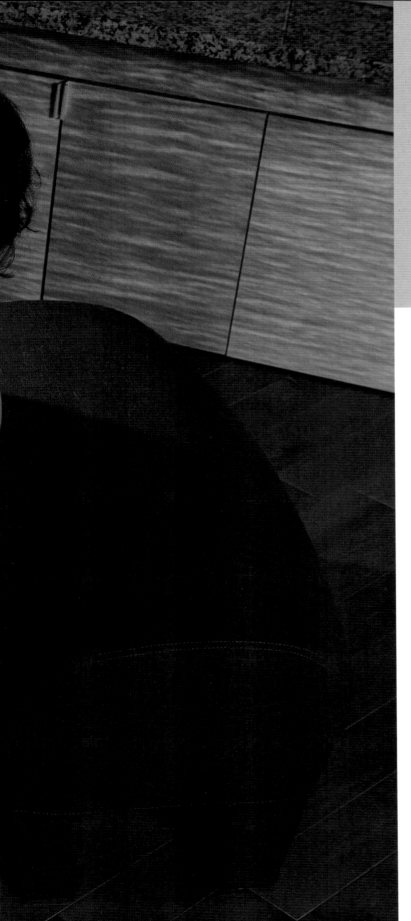

" Real talk "

From Laura: "There was a great oral sex-film moment that transfixed my mother's generation: Jon Voight in *Coming Home* (1978), playing a Vietnam vet paralyzed from the waist down, performing cunnilingus on Jane Fonda, wife of an officer who would kill himself at the end of the film. The message was implicit: The husband committed suicide because he was less a man in bed than a cripple.

"My generation has Chloe Sevigny in that infamous cunnilingus scene with Vincent Gallo in *The Brown Bunny* (2003). It's more explicit. Yes, hotter. Yet it lacks the edginess of the older film—and certainly misses the sacramental aspect of cunnilingus. Voight worshipped at her altar. Gallo—Uh, no. He was just in it for him self."

Technique Tip

SWALLOWING

This is definitely extra credit. Swallowing is not really difficult—and he will love you for doing it. A man feels totally accepted and loved when a woman swallows his semen. You can control the depth of oral penetration via the ring and seal and influence the timing by pressing his perineum.

Position yourself so that his ejaculate will shoot straight down your throat. An easy way of doing this: Lie on your back with your head off the bed. Your mouth and throat will form a smooth line. Have him straddle your face for the elegant finish to a perfect blow job.

Two golden rules of fellatio:

No head bobbing—it just looks

silly—and keep your tongue

moving all the time.

The Basic Black Dress of Blow Jobs

- Kiss and lick his inner thighs while pulling down ever so slightly on his scrotum. With your finger pads, scratch his testicles. Put his balls carefully into your mouth one at a time. Roll them around. Then, again ever so gently, pull them down with your mouth.

- While you're attending to his balls, run your fingers lovingly up and down the shaft of his penis.

- Get into a comfortable position, kneeling at his side on the bed or at a right angle to his body or kneeling between his legs. Or you can bring him down to the edge of the bed and kneel on the floor. Wet your lips and be sure that they cover your teeth. Run your tongue around the head of his penis to moisten it.

- Hold the base of his penis firmly in one hand. With the other hand, you can form a circle with your thumb and forefinger—what sex expert Lou Paget calls "the ring and the seal"—to elongate your mouth and prevent him from going in farther than you would like. Use that hand in a twisting motion as you fellate him. Or, if his erection is not firm, you can use both hands (wrapped around the shaft) in an upward twist stroke.

- Circle the head with your tongue in a swirling motion, and then work your tongue in long strokes up and down his shaft. Now back to the head.

- Follow the ridge of the corona with your tongue while working the shaft with your hands, the penis sandwiched between them—unless, of course, you want to keep that ring and seal in place.

- Strum the frenulum with your tongue. Lick the raphe.

- Make eye contact with him from time to time.

- Do at least ten or twenty seconds of this showy move: Repeatedly pull his penis into your mouth, then push it out, using suction?while keeping that tongue in motion.

- Go back to the head. Swirl your tongue around it. Tongue the corona. Suck the head. Repeat, repeat, repeat.

- Follow his lead if he pulls back from stimulation. He knows that he will reach orgasm sooner than he would like if you don't stop. Take his hand and put it against your vagina. Let him stimulate you until his excitement subsides a bit.

- But if you want him to come, apply gentle pressure with thumb or finger to his perineum.

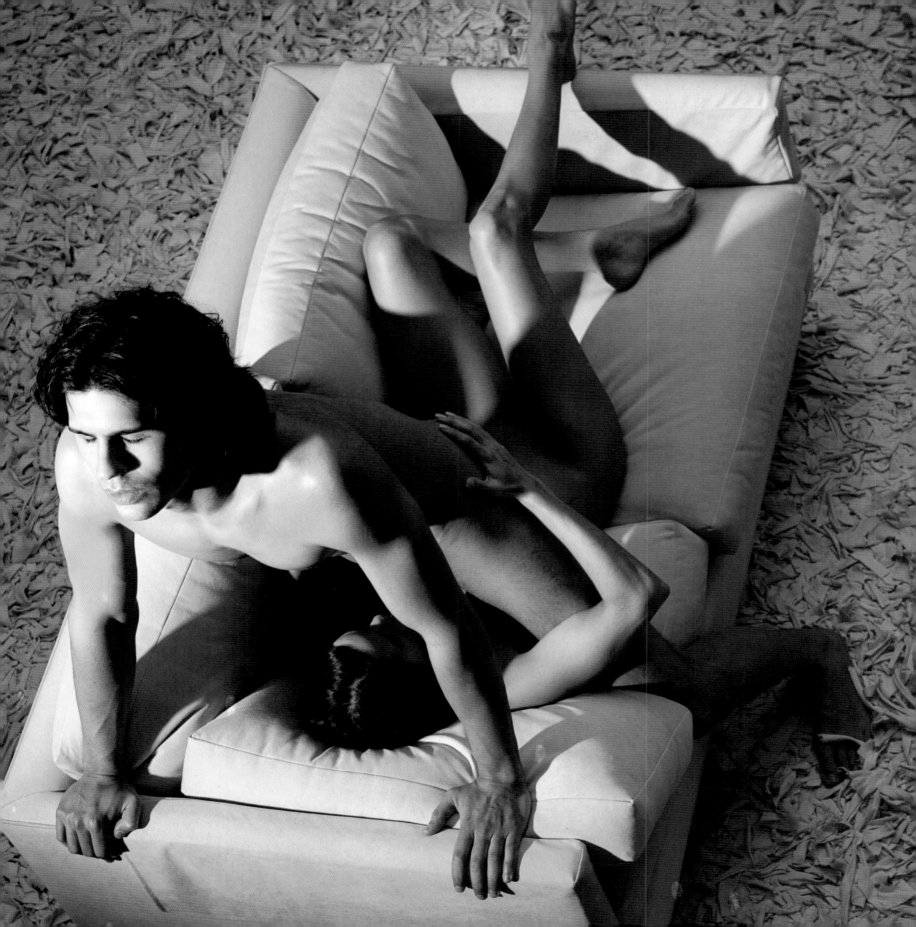

A COUPLE'S STORY

This is not a politically correct story. Angie met Donald at a major urban university where he was a professor and she was a student. The subject was biology, tangentially related to human sexuality, but related nonetheless.

"I was a few years older than most of the students," Angie says, "and he was a very young professor. Yes, we were both married to other people. And, no, it wasn't right. But the attraction was too strong to deny."

Their affair began with stolen kisses in his office, progressed to playing "footsie" under the table of a local pub where they met for lunch, and reached a glorious high point on an orange chenille bedspread at a nearby motel.

"I'd received oral sex before," she says, "but not from anyone who really knew how to perform cunnilingus. The first time he did it, I remember feeling the heat building behind my clitoris. I was so hot, I felt like I might boil over. Writhing under his tongue, I began panting and gasping. At one point the tip of his tongue was moving so fast around my clitoris that it was like being ravished by a hundred butterflies with whirring wings.

"I came! I had a big explosive orgasm. He stroked my labia and put his fingers inside me and held his tongue over my clitoris without moving for what seemed an eternity but must have been a minute or two. Then he repeated his amazing feat and gave me another orgasm.

"My whole life changed that day.

"I knew I couldn't go back to a husband who gargled following cunnilingus. My marriage dragged on for several months, but it was effectively over that day."

Donald made promises to leave his wife, but he never did. Angie was crushed and broke off the relationship. Years later, however, she looks back at him with only love and gratitude.

"He was my sexual awakening," she says. "I knew I had to have that kind of loving and I have never settled for less."

The man she will marry soon is, she says, a "consummate oral lover." When she told him her story, he understood completely. In that moment, she knew she'd found the love of her life.

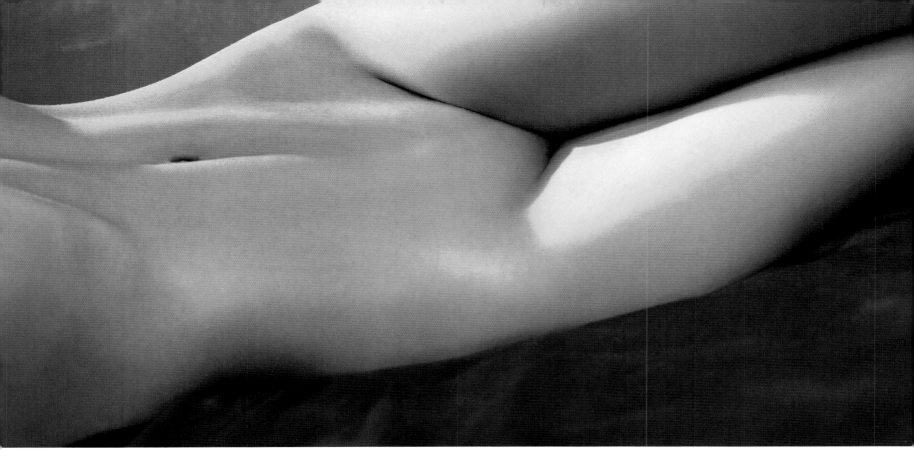

Cunnilingus

Most men love performing cunnilingus almost as much as they do receiving fellatio. In fact, many men report that they want to give, but their partners shy away from receiving oral sex. Surprisingly, women in their twenties are generally less assertive about getting their oral needs met than older women are. They expect to perform oral sex but not necessarily to receive it.

Both the giving and the receiving of oral sex are essential skills.

Three things to remember about pleasing her orally: Use soft, gentle strokes, paying attention to her cues for more (or even less) pressure. Don't imitate the exaggerated tongue flicking that you see in porn films. It looks great but isn't that effective. And don't go straight for her clitoris.

But she still says, "No, thanks"?

If she's still reluctant to receive cunnilingus, there are things you can do to change her mind.

- Get her to the verge of orgasm via foreplay. When she's begging for penetration, use your tongue instead. Nothing like an orgasm for showing a woman she likes oral sex after all.

- Assume that her previous partners just didn't know what they were doing. Make sure *you* do. Practice your licking and sucking techniques on her lips and the tip of her tongue. Pay attention to her responses until you have fine-tuned your mouth moves to suit her exactly. Whisper in her ear that you want nothing more than to take that magic south.

- If she's a confident, secure, adventurous woman, ask her to explain *why*. Address her concerns. Get her to strike a deal: She has to give you three chances before ruling cunnilingus out again.

- This power move can actually take a shy woman through her wall of reserve. Why? Because you're giving her the power in a highly symbolic way. Kneel before her. Knead her buttocks softly as you bury your face in her vulva. Inhale deeply, sigh happily. Begin licking from her knees up to her inner thighs. Manually stimulate her labia, vulva, vagina, and finally clitoris as you give her thighs little sucking kisses and work your lips up to their goal. (Just look at those numbers curled into each other!) There are two basic ways of doing it: lying side by side, mouths to genitals, or one partner straddling the other, again mouths to genitals. Either partner can be on top. Mutual oral stimulation is more exciting in theory than in practice. When you are highly aroused, it is hard to concentrate on your own technique. Neither partner is likely to be as adept as when working alone.

"*Cunnilingus is the best thing you can do for a woman. It makes her feel sexy and loved. You may have the smallest penis on the planet, but if you do this well, you are a fabulous lover to her.*"

— Bob Berkowitz, Ph.D.
Broadcast journalist
and author

Going Down Gracefully

- Start at the top. Stroke, massage, nibble, suck, kiss, lick, and otherwise tease and tantalize her body, avoiding her genitals until she is aroused.

- Pay special attention to her breasts. Massage her areolae with flat, open palms, then play with the nipples as you lick and kiss slowly down a line from her navel to the edge of her pubic hair.

- Lick the line of flesh between her pelvis and her thighs. Kiss and lick up and down one inner thigh to the area behind her knee. Now the other.

- Get into a position comfortable for both of you. She may lean against pillows either with legs open, knees bent, feet flat, or with legs outstretched and open to a V. You can lie or kneel between her legs or come in from the side and wrap a leg around your shoulder. Or she can straddle your face and lower her clitoris to your mouth. A lot of women love this position because it puts them in charge.

- Gently part her labia. Holding them open, lift the clitoral hood. If her clitoris is well back inside the hood, gently run your fingers along the side of the hood to expose the clitoris. (You may have to keep one hand in this position until she reaches orgasm.)

- Lick the delicate tissue along the sides and above and below her clitoris in long, broad strokes of the tongue.

- Experiment with your tongue strokes.

- Put your lips around the sides of her clitoris. Hold them in a pursed position as you gently suck. Alternate the sucking with licking of the surrounding tissues.

- If she likes direct stimulation of the clitoris, lick and suck it.

- When she is nearing orgasm, cover the clitoral area with your mouth. Suck around the sides of her clitoris. Stimulate her labia with your hand or stroke her inner thighs or tease her nipples—or alternate these stimuli. But do not move your mouth until she has reached orgasm unless you plan to bring her to orgasm via intercourse.

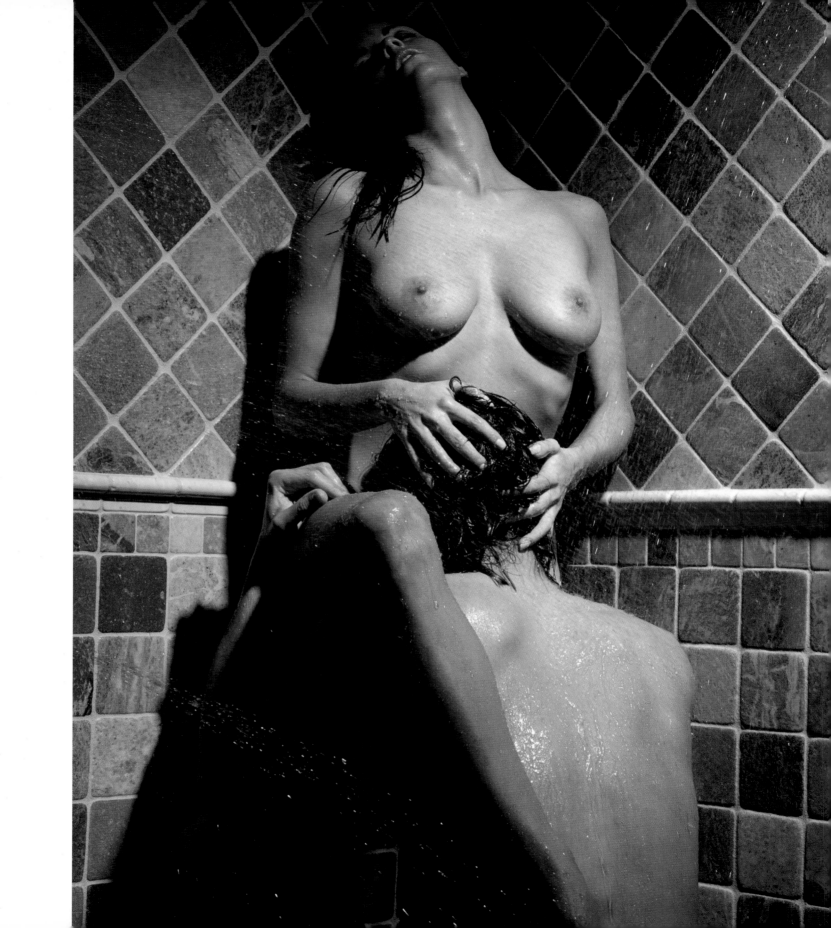

FANCY STROKES

For extra credit, perfect these strokes:

The Flick. Using only the tip of your tongue—no broad strokes!—flick back and forth rapidly along the clitoral shaft. When she is approaching orgasm, flick back and forth across the top of the clitoris. (Caution: This is too much direct stimulation for some women.)

The Velvet No. Use this technique on a multiorgasmic woman who likes a stronger touch after her first orgasm. Put the tip of your tongue against the shaft of her clitoris and hold it steady. Move your head back and forth as if you were saying, "No, no, no." The key to this move is holding your tongue steady while you move your head.

"Real talk"

"Josh never got the tongue action right when he performed cunnilingus," says Amanda. "One day we were manually stimulating each other. He moved his hand from my pussy to his cock and started pumping it. I got the message; that's how he likes it pumped. I took my hand away from my clitoris, put it into his mouth. He sucked my juices. Then I kissed him, pulled back, and flicked the tip of my tongue rapidly back and forth across the tip of his tongue.

"He got the message."

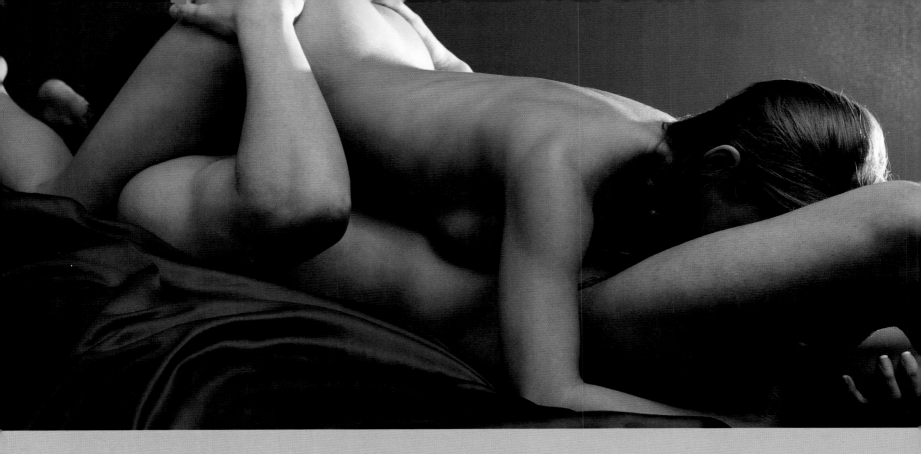

69

To make the 69 work better, take turns stimulating each other when you've reached that high point. When he is active, she can hold his penis in her mouth or even outside her mouth, where it will be stimulated by her hot breath. When she is actively stimulating him, he can rest his mouth on her vulva so his hot interlude, rather than his tongue, tickles her.

Doing it this way sustains the arousal period—and keeps one partner from accidentally biting the other.

Technique Tip

While performing oral sex, vary the temperature of your mouth. Start with normal body temperature. Then, using your hand to stimulate your partner, fill your mouth with ice cubes. Wait until your tongue is numb before spitting out the ice. Apply your frozen assets to his genitals. That will feel like a jolt of sexual electricity to him.

After a few minutes, when your oral temperature is back to normal, repeat the procedure, this time filling your mouth with a hot drink.

This method of alternating temperatures restores erection in most men and can prolong the arousal phase for some. Others say they have more intense orgasms when heat and ice are applied.

Can oral sex save a marriage? Make a man or a woman fall in love with you?

Maybe. Men and women who love oral sex believe in its power. More than one wealthy man in the public eye reputedly left his wife for a woman who performed fellatio with passion and skill.

But can you teach your partner to do it well?

Yes—if he or she wants to learn.

In the Western world, at this point in history, oral sex is a nearly indispensable part of lovemaking. Cunnilingus is the one sure path (aside from the vibrator) to female orgasm. Fellatio is every man's heart's desire.

You can upgrade your lover's performance skills by:

KEEPING YOUR CRITICISM CONSTRUCTIVE

An example of constructive criticism: "Honey, I really love it when you lick and suck my clitoris, but it's so sensitive when I'm aroused—and you *do* arouse me!—could you please be a little more gentle?"

That is so much better than "Ouch! You're hurting me! Don't do that!"

Another example of constructive criticism: Put your hand over her hand as she holds the base of your penis while performing fellatio. Squeeze. Show her the intensity you want by demonstrating the grip you need—rather than shoving your penis into her mouth.

And only when she is holding you tightly do you say, "Please, please, more, harder, faster, please—take me deeper, please."

SHOWING MORE, TELLING LESS

Mutual masturbation can be a tutorial on how you like your genitals handled. If you masturbate side by side while kissing and caressing each other, the tutorial is even more useful—because it adds mouth moves. Let him (or her) see the connection between the way you caress your own genitals and the way you use your lips and the tip of your tongue on your lover's mouth and tongue.

BRINGING IN AN OUTSIDE SOURCE

Read aloud to your lover an outstanding and detailed description of oral sex—as part of foreplay. Don't introduce these segments by saying, "Here's how you should do it." Instead ask, "Isn't this hot?"

Keep erotic reading material at your bedside. If the first reading doesn't produce the longed-for results, maybe the second or third will. Some videos and DVDs are useful, too—if they show a realistic performance of oral sex.

If you can comfortably say it, then say, "Oh, look at that. How do you suppose he [or she] does *that*?"

"Real talk"

From Dave: "Most women aren't very good at performing oral sex. They just don't do it long enough. Or they haven't figured out how to get around the gag reflex. Nothing spoils your pleasure like hearing a woman choking on your penis. When a woman is good at it, she's usually very good. Ah, a woman who knows how to love a man's penis is truly God's gift to man. It feels like she's performing a sacrament on your body."

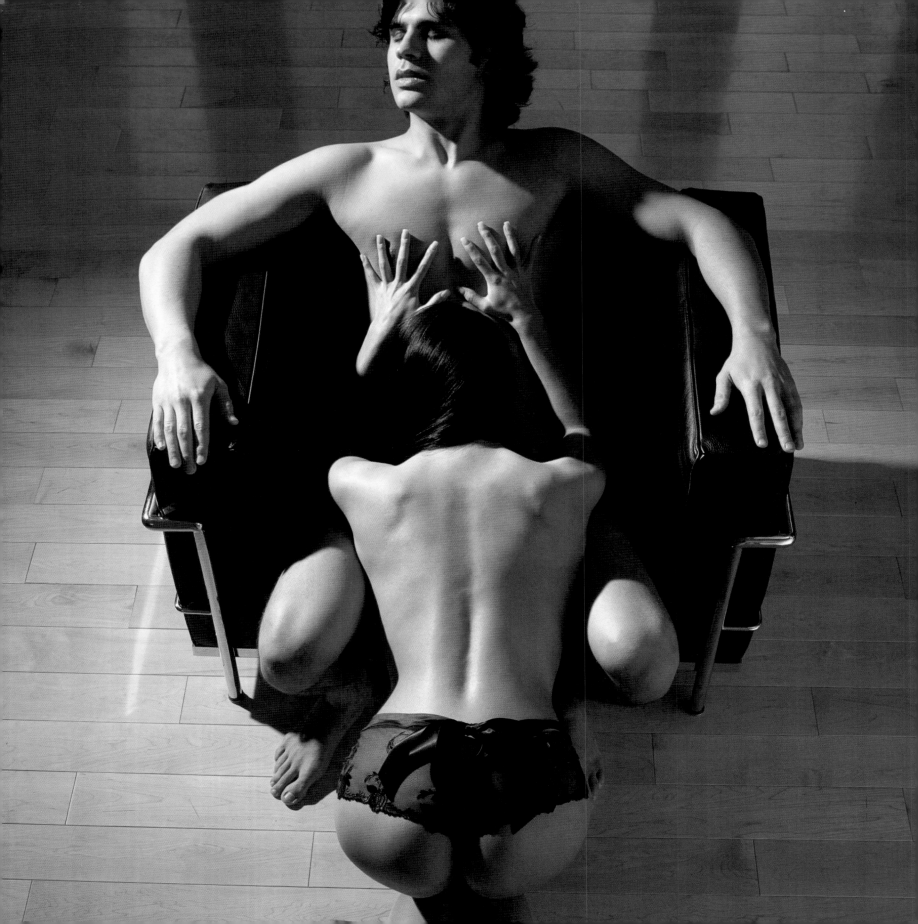

A COUPLE'S STORY

"I worship Robert's penis," Sharon says. "A little penis worship is good for the soul. Every woman should worship her man this way."

Robert is quick to add that he worships her vagina, too.

On a trip to India several years ago, this couple discovered the yoni (vagina) and the lingam (penis), objects of fetish and worship typically made of stone or glass. They bought several, made a little altar in their bedroom, and began reading about the history of sacred sexuality.

"I have always loved Robert's penis," she says. "It is a thing of beauty, like an ebony sculpture. I love the way he smells and tastes, too. The lingams in our bedroom inspired me to love his penis even more.

"I like to fellate him to orgasm at least once a week. My favorite position is kneeling before him."

Occasionally Sharon indulges her enthusiasm for Robert's penis outside their home.

"We were having a drink in the lobby bar of a Manhattan hotel," she says, "when I put my hand in his lap and felt his magnificence stirring. I played with him through his slacks until he was having trouble sitting still.

"He pulled my face close and whispered in my ear, 'Let's go.'"

They paid the check. As she was walking toward the door (and heading home to their apartment), he took her by the shoulders, turned her gently around, and steered her into the elevator. They went up to the twelfth floor. Why twelve? No one else got off on that floor. At the end of the hallway, he told her to kneel and unzipped his pants.

"It was thrilling," she says. "I took his penis into my mouth as he held my head in his hands. I sucked and licked and in a very short time, I tasted his hot, sweet cum. He helped me to my feet and zipped up his pants just as someone opened a door down the hall."

If a woman wants to see the extent of her erotic power over a man, she should perform oral sex on him. Not only will he be physically thrilled, but eternally grateful.

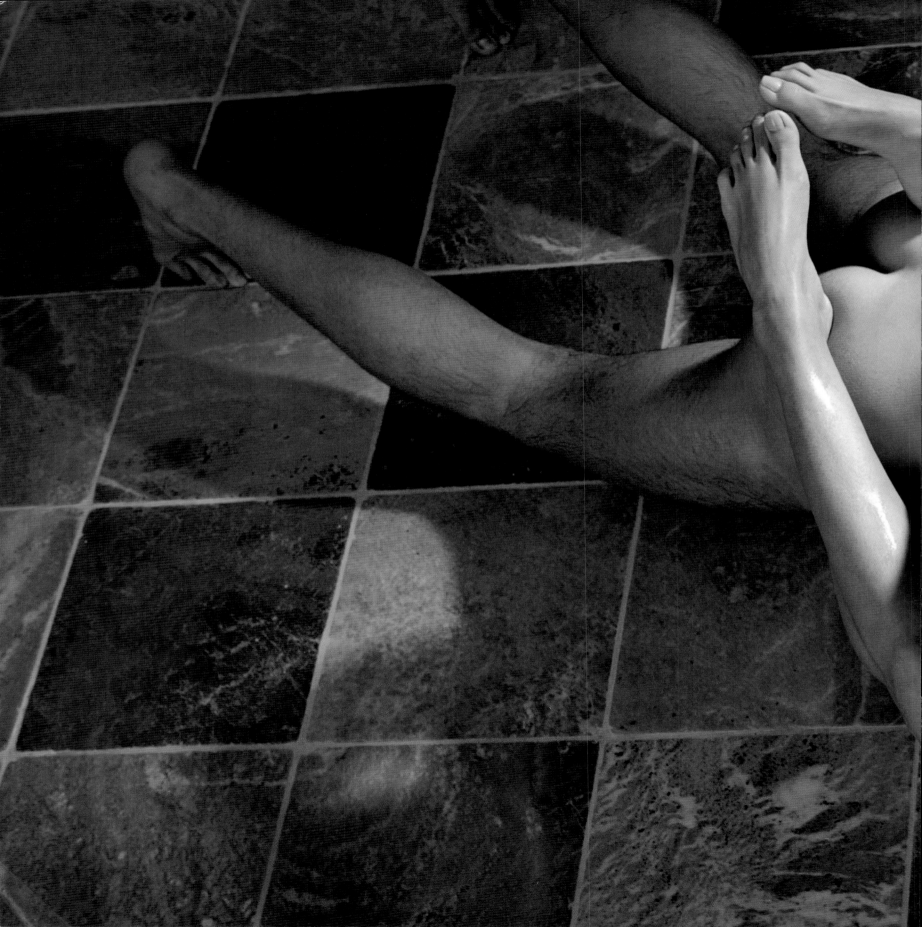

4

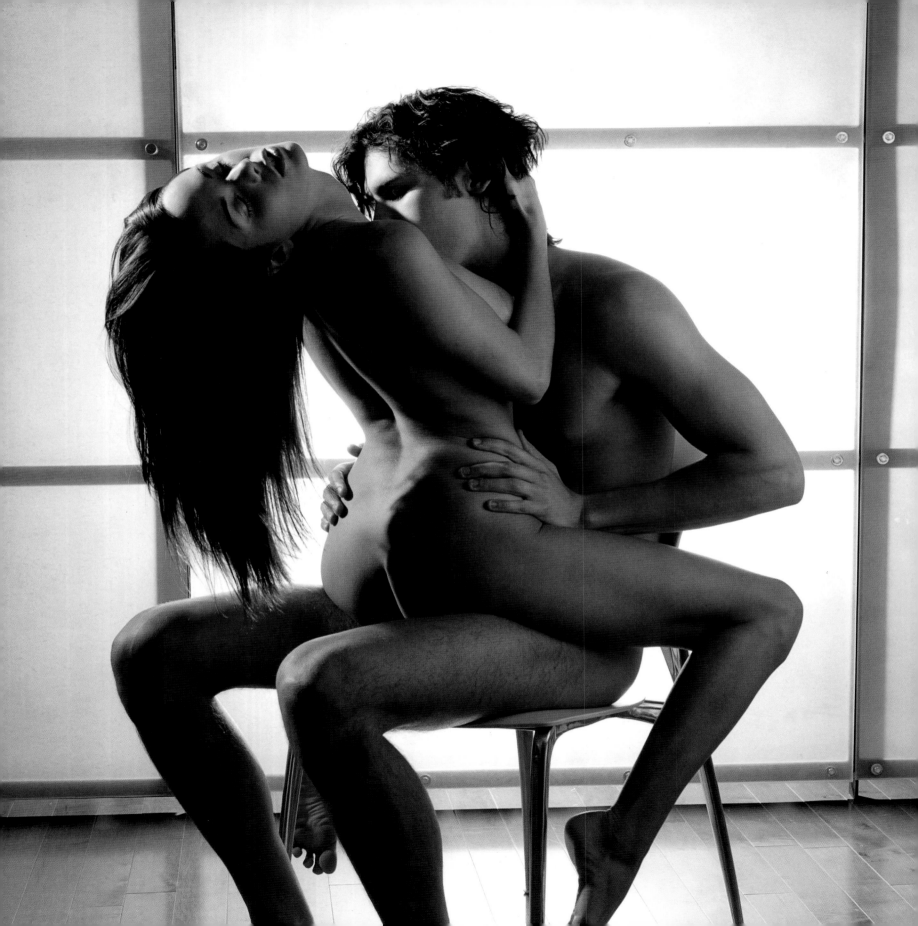

THE POSITIONS AND TECHNIQUES

———

"There are three 'feel good' standards for any intercourse position:

comfort, visual stimulation, and arousal, his and hers. I never say

any one position is 'the best' or something a couple 'must do.'

What is good for them depends on how their bodies work together,

what they find arousing, what is comfortable for them.

Nobody ever had great sex in a position that didn't feel good."

— Prokash Kothari, M.D.
Famed Mumbai sexologist

THERE ARE SIX basic intercourse positions: woman on top (female superior), man on top (missionary), rear entry, side by side, sitting, and standing. Every couple should be fluent in the basic positions. You may have a favorite position with your partner, likely based on the way your bodies fit and move together. Every position, however, can be adapted to meet your needs—and one of those needs is variety. Bodies also change with injury, pregnancy, illness, weight gain or loss, and, of course, age. What did work once may not work as well today.

On the other hand, some positions that you didn't like could be in the "oh, yes" column now. As women pass the age of thirty and become more sexually confident, for example, they may love being on top, whereas they formerly felt too exposed in that position. And as men age a bit, they are more relaxed about letting her be in charge some of the time.

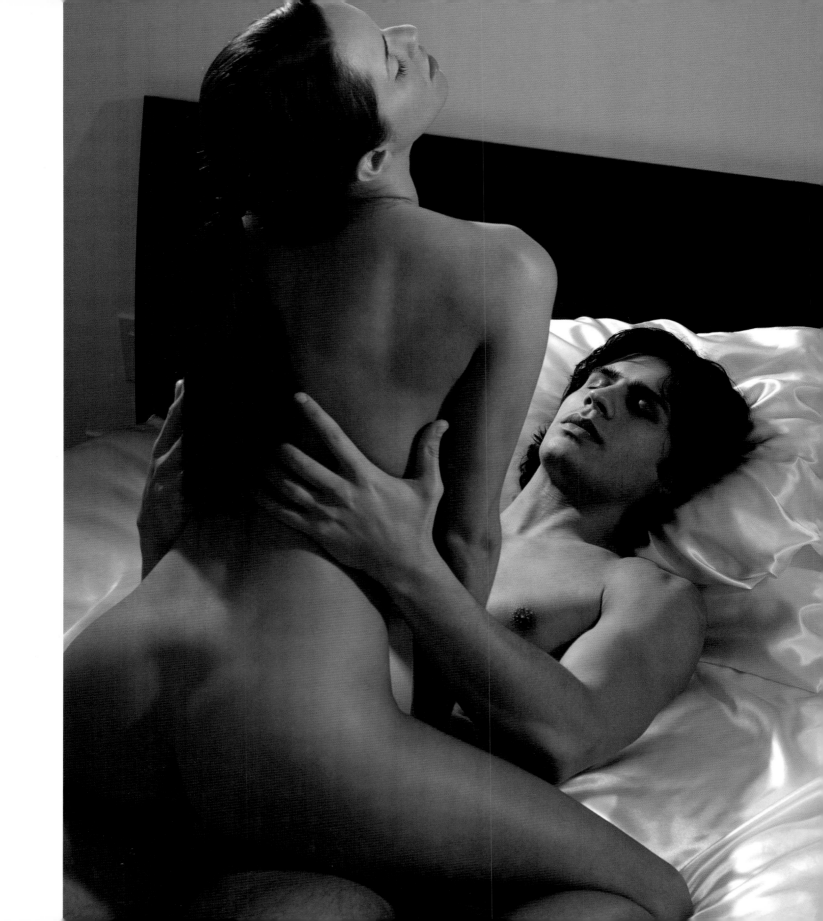

THE BASICS
OF THE BASIC SIX

Female Superior Position

This is generally considered the most favorable position for female orgasm, because she has the freedom to stroke her clitoris during intercourse—and to control the angle and depth of penetration and the speed of thrusting.

HIS BONUS: visual stimulation.

THE POSITION: She squats or sits astride him as he lies on his back. Her legs are bent at the knees, one on either side of his body. She may lean forward or backward, using her hands for support, or sit upright, keeping both hands free. Or she may straddle him facing his feet, not his head, in the "reverse cowgirl" position.

Technique Tip

THE FEMALE SUPERIOR TWIST

This little adaptation of an old favorite puts a new spin on the concept of getting it her way. He lies on his back. She straddles him, facing his feet, not his head. He raises one leg, bent at the knee, foot on the bed. She angles her body so that she is riding his penis at the same time she is grinding her pelvis against his raised thigh.

Slow motion for him—but double action for her.

"Real talk"

"My first husband was very macho," says Jessica. "He would let me be on top only occasionally as a 'special treat.' I was young when I married him, so I didn't know what a jerk he was until I left him and met other men. My second husband is a real man. Sometimes he takes me in a very masterful way. Other times he is happy to let me ride him. I love being on top. I come faster that way, but I also love the position because he enjoys watching me so much."

Technique Tip

THE OVAL TRACK

A sizzling move, the Oval Track looks as good to him as it feels to her.

Simply move in an oval track rather than a straightforward up-and-down pattern. Imagine you are circumscribing an oval with your body, with the downstroke at one end of the oval and the upstroke at the other. Lean slightly forward as you push down on his penis, stimulating your clitoris. Pull up and move slightly backward on the upstroke, stimulating your G-spot.

Technique Tip

THE CORKSCREW TWIST

Sit on top of him, insert him, and lean forward, lifting yourself three-quarters of the way up his penis. Put your hands on his shoulders for balance. Then move your pelvis to the right and push yourself down at the same time. Pull back up and move your pelvis to the left as you push down again. Go back and forth like this for several cycles.

Add a PC (Kegel directions on page 36) flex to the move. Tighten your PC muscle on the downward push, and then relax it while coming up.

Or, if you are flexible, do the twist while bending backward with your hands resting on his knees.

A variation of the corkscrew twist is for her to face away from the man and lean forward with her hands on his knees, while he sits upright on a couch, chair, or bed. This position not only provides deeper penetration for her, but a different and stimulating view for him.

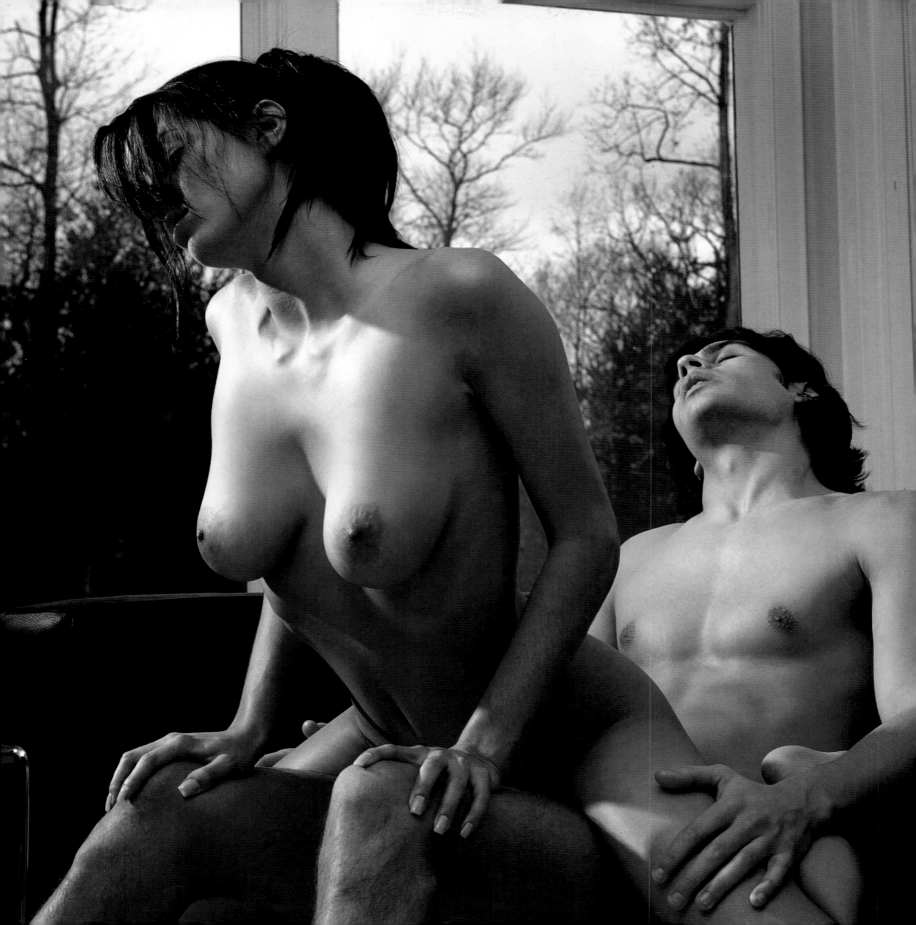

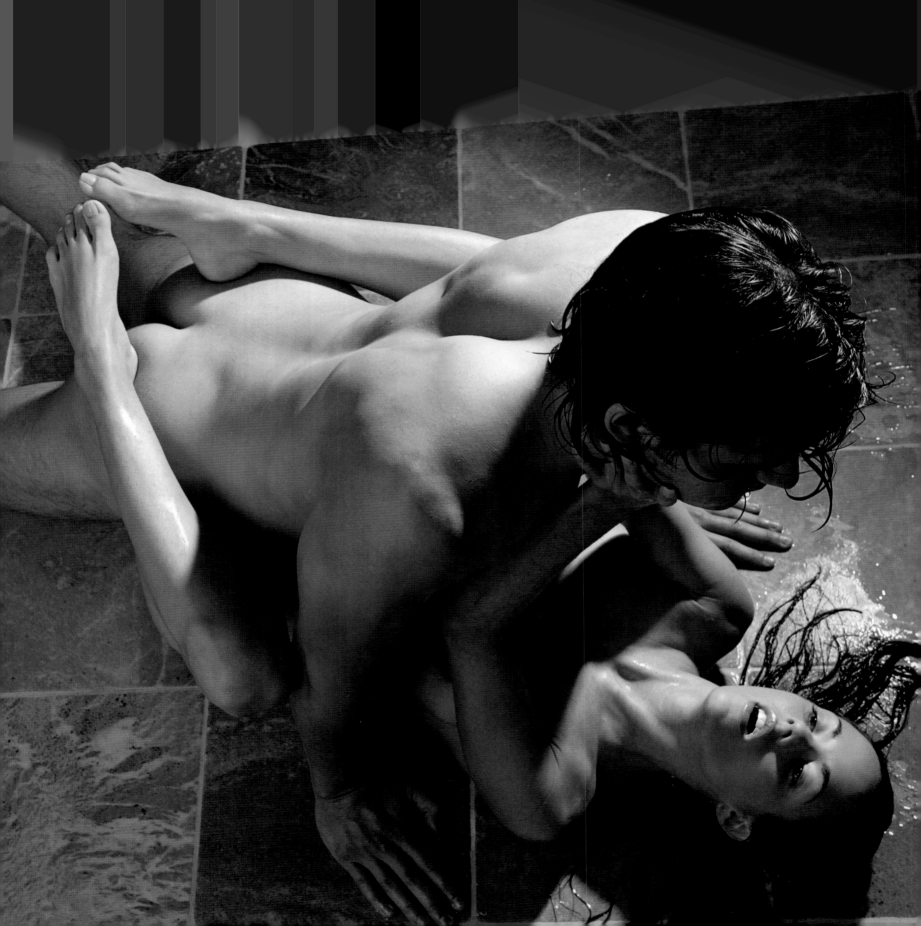

The Missionary Position

According to legend, Pacific Islanders named this position after the missionaries who had sex only this way. The position has been unfairly maligned ever since. It's a great one for hard thrusting and emotional contact.

HER BONUS: Many women love this position as much as men do because it combines penetration and intimacy.

THE POSITION: She lies on her back with her legs slightly parted. He lies on top of her, supporting his weight at least partially with his hands or elbows. They can lessen or increase the depth of penetration by putting pillows under the small of her back or her buttocks or wrapping her legs around his waist or placing her feet on his shoulders.

"For many women, lying in the missionary position

with a few pillows under their butts provides

the perfect pelvis tilt for G-spot stimulation—and orgasm."

— Laura Berman, M.D.
Talk-show host and author

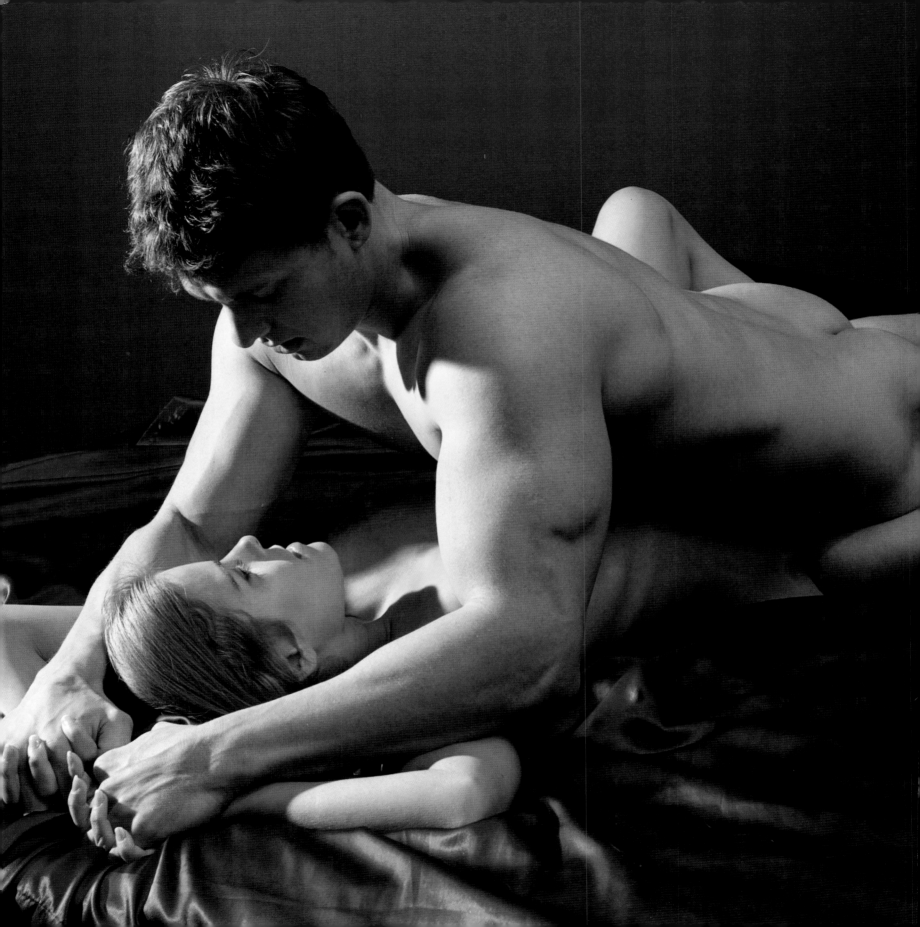

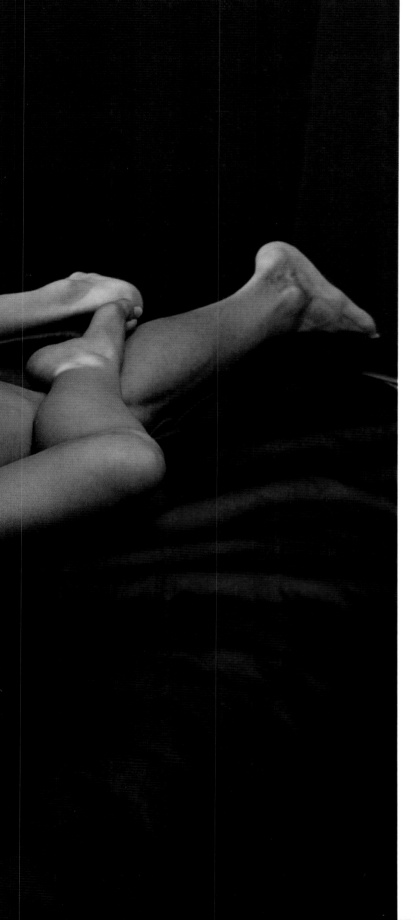

Technique Tip

THE CAT OR COITAL ALIGNMENT TECHNIQUE

Want an old-fashioned simultaneous orgasm in the missionary position?

Sex experts have been saying for years that striving for a simultaneous orgasm with your partner is not realistic. They are certainly right about that. Some women, however, are desperate to achieve this. Often they are the same women who have difficulty reaching orgasm at all during intercourse. The CAT was developed by an Australian male psychotherapist to fulfill the desire of these women.

She lies on her back. He lies on top of her with his full weight on top of her so that his pelvis is higher than her clitoris. She wraps her legs around his thighs, resting her ankles on his calves.

The key to success: Move only your pelvises in a steady rhythm, which neither speeds up nor slows down until orgasm is achieved by both lovers.

She leads on the upward stroke, pushing his pelvis backward while he simultaneously provides a counter-pressure on her clitoris with the shaft of his penis. He leads on the downward stroke, pushing her pelvis downward while she provides a resistant counter-pressure by pressing her clitoris against the base of his penis.

The cautionary proviso: This position is not for everyone. If he is a lot larger than she is, she will be uncomfortable, at the least.

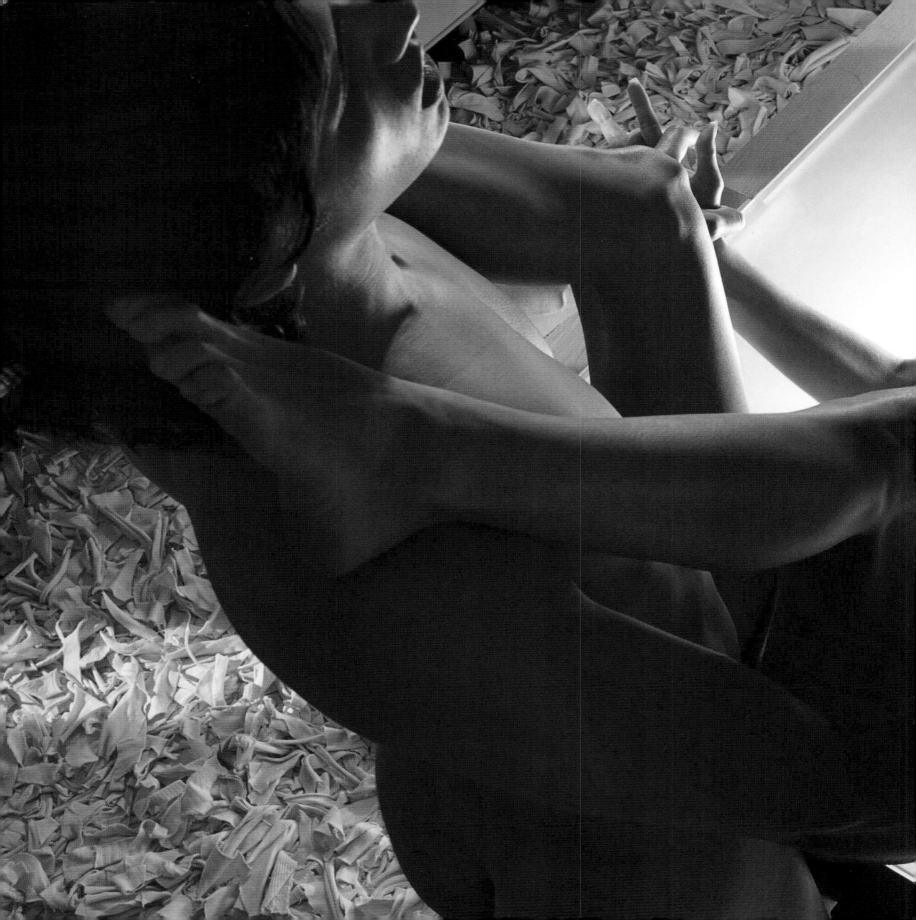

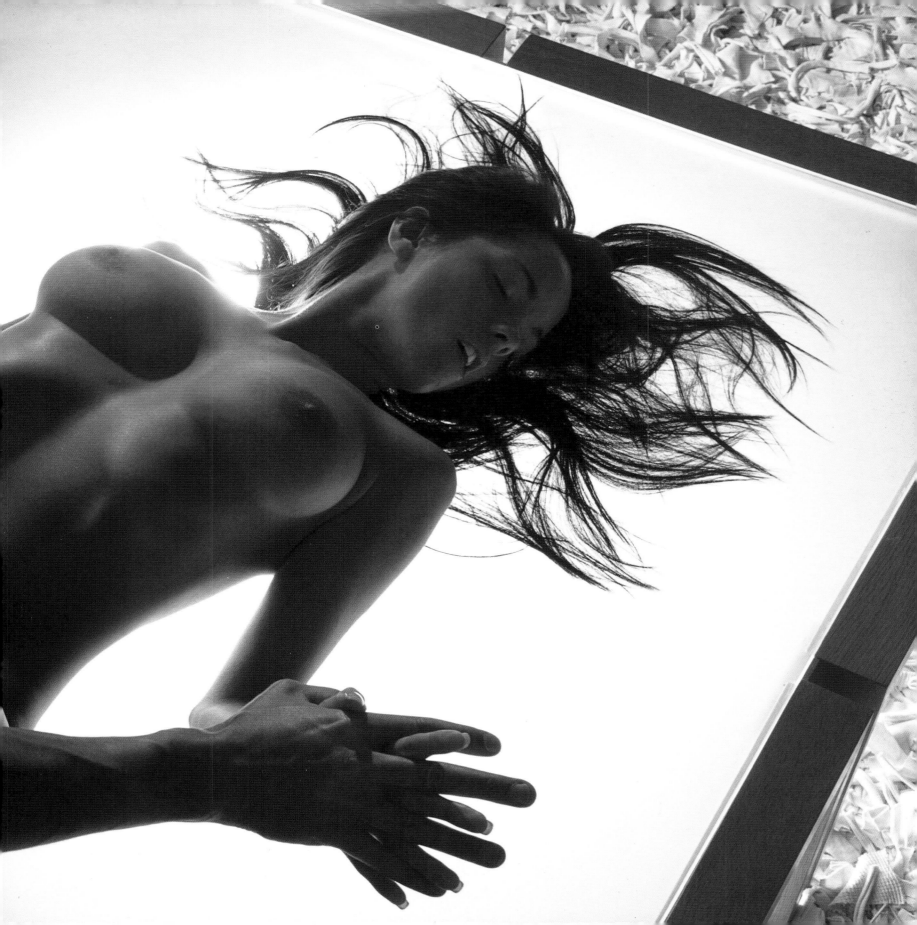

THE HEAD TRICK

Intercourse in the missionary position can lead to ejaculation for him faster than he—or she—would like.

You want to slow down without slowing her down. How do you do it?

When you feel very aroused during intercourse—but you haven't reached that point of ejaculatory inevitability—withdraw your penis so that only the head remains inside her vagina. Remain motionless for ten to thirty seconds. Resume thrusting slowly.

You can use this move two, three, even multiple times during intercourse.

An Easier Simultaneous Orgasm

A generation or two ago, women believed that a simultaneous orgasm was the ultimate in lovemaking—so they faked theirs in time with his.

Now we know it's a nice intimacy bonus, but we don't have to fake to get it.

If the CAT is not your style, try the following:

1. STRETCH OUT FOREPLAY. Let the "faster" partner (probably him) focus more oral and manual attention on the "slower" partner. Don't begin intercourse until the two of you are in sync. You know the signs: panting, sweating, asking for it in a shaky voice. Place your hands on each other's lower backs or thighs so you can easily communicate the necessary commands, slower or faster. If one of you is almost there and the other isn't, he (or she) should pull back. The "faster" partner kisses and caresses his (or her) lover.

   Maintaining eye contact will help you communicate better.

2. FORGET "LADIES FIRST." He usually gives her the first orgasm via cunnilingus. But this time he stops oral stimulation when she is on the brink of orgasm. She gives him the manual or oral stimulation he needs to "catch up." They start intercourse at the same place—on high. And they keep their hands on each other's hips so they can quickly indicate faster or slower.

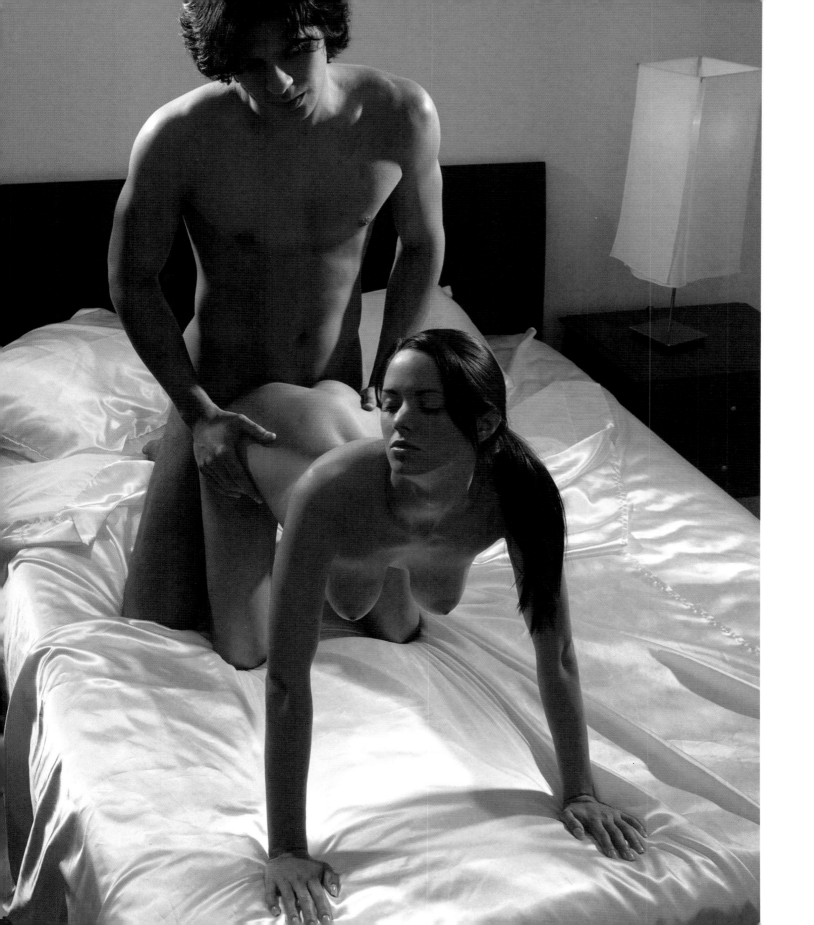

Rear Entry Position

Women love this or they don't. Men generally do. Rear entry facilitates deeper penetration than the other basic positions. Women who experience G-spot orgasms are more likely to do so in this position than in any other.

BONUS: It can almost satisfy a man's desire for anal sex because he has the same view: woman in submissive posture, ass alluringly exposed. And the lack of face-to-face contact makes it easier for one or both partners to fantasize—something we all need to do now and then—or to make love if they are angry with each other.

THE POSITION: She is on all fours with him kneeling behind her. She can change the angle of penetration by lowering her chest to the bed. That also leaves a hand free for stimulating her clitoris.

Technique Tip

SIMULATED ANAL SEX

He wants it tonight. You don't want to go there. Let him insert a finger or two into your anus. Do it in the rear entry position, but spike the experience for him by talking through a hot anal-intercourse scenario. Jazz it up by playing a DVD or video featuring anal intercourse.

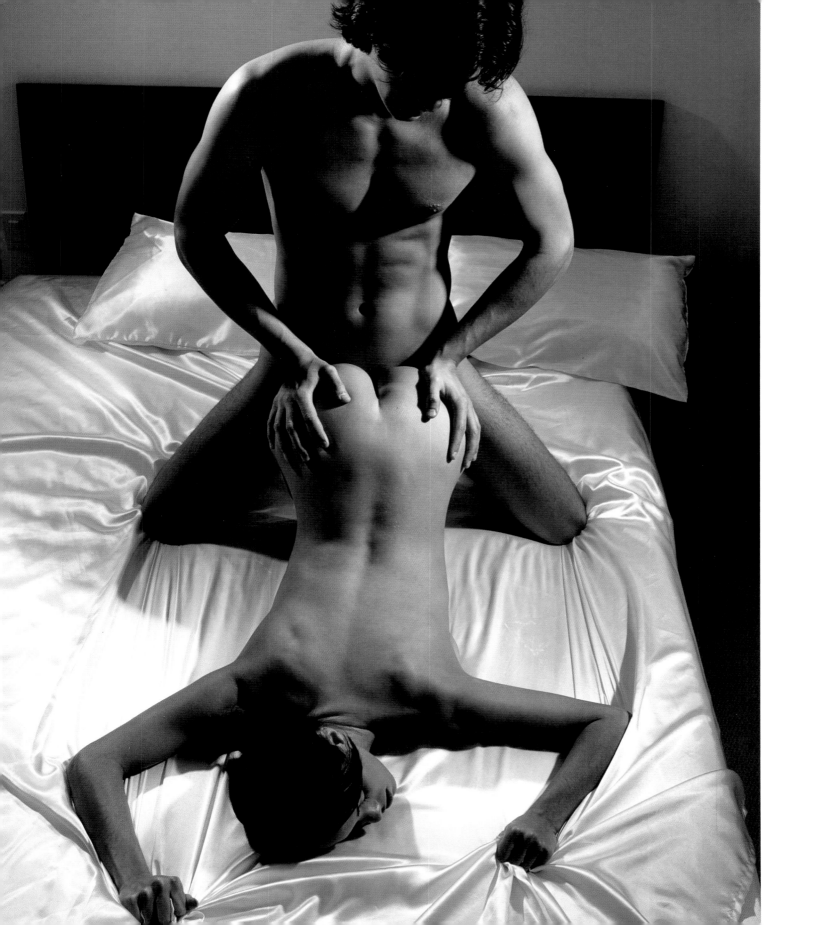

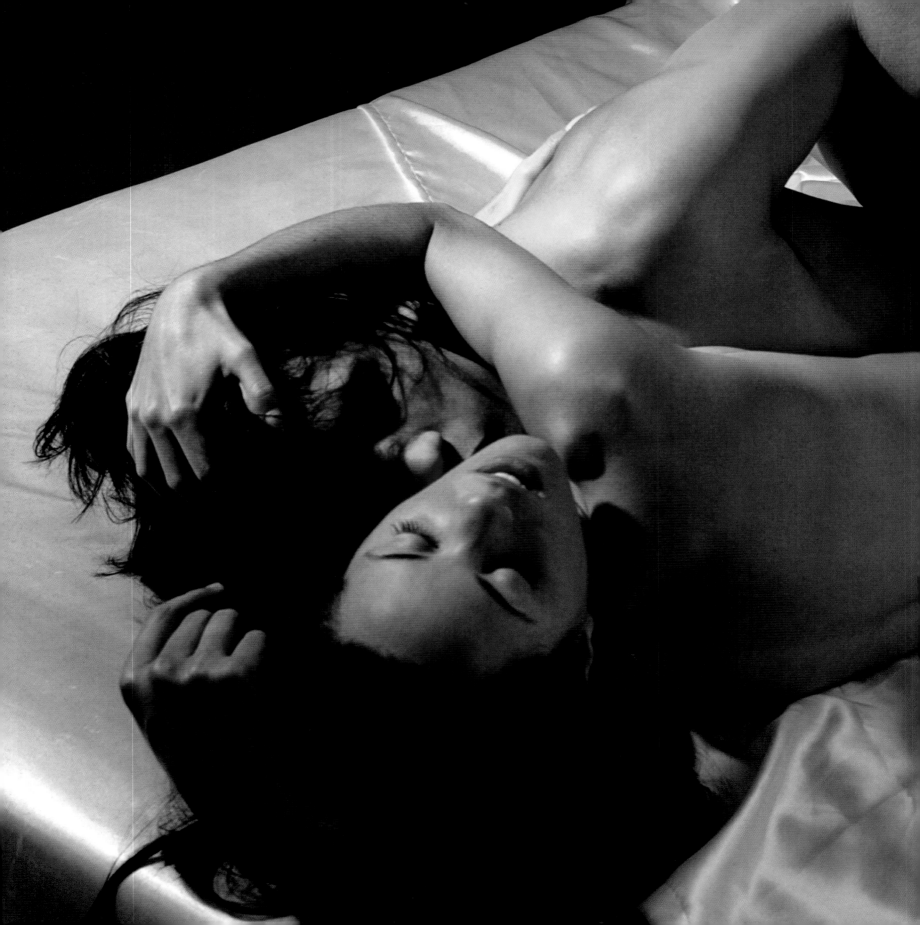

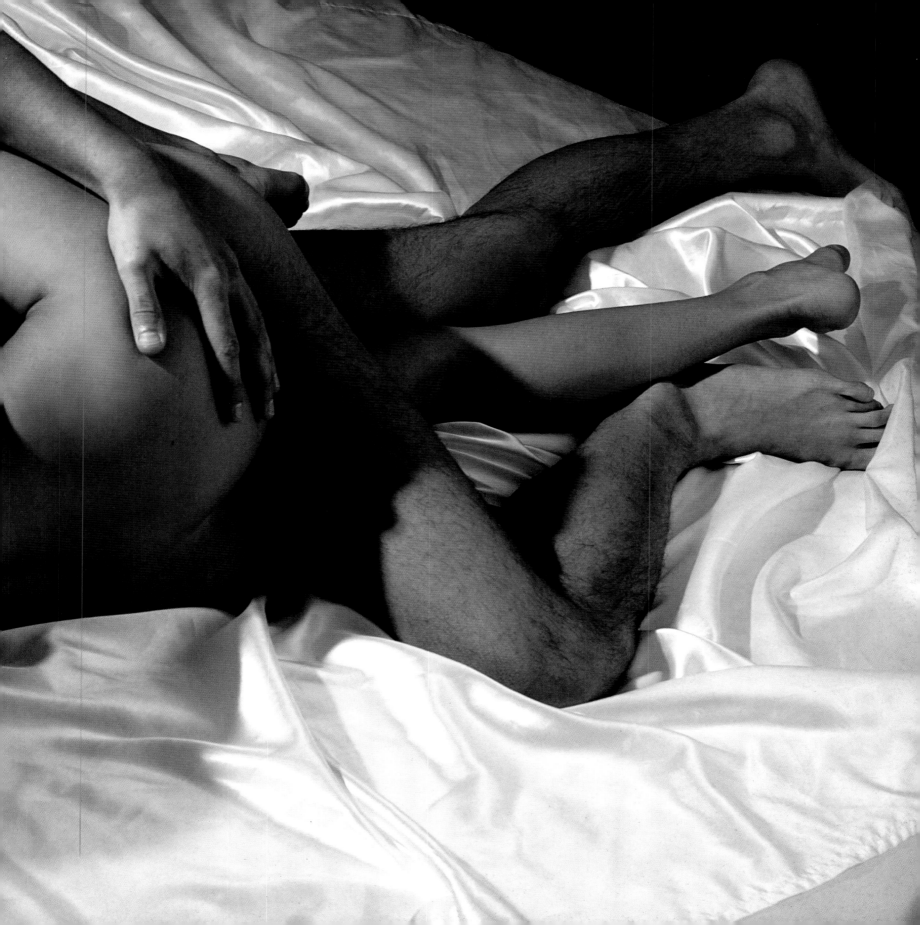

Side by Side (or Spoon) Position

Penetration is limited in the spoon position. No wonder the French call it *la paresseuse*, meaning "the lazy way."

BONUS: It's a perfect position for the couple who are "too tired" but want to have sex. And it works in late pregnancy when almost nothing else does.

THE POSITION: He faces her back. Her buttocks are angled against him as he puts one leg between hers. Or she can lie half on her back, half on her side, drawing up one leg.

"STUFF" AND SPOON

He has only a semierection, but you both want to have sex?

In the spoon position, his front to your back, insert his semierect penis into your vagina. With fingers splayed downward, use one hand to hold the penis in place between your thumb and first finger, forming a V around the base, the flat of your palm caressing the shaft. Massage his perineum. A perineum massage will give many men an erection. Use the other hand to stroke your clitoris. Maintain a slow but steady intercourse motion.

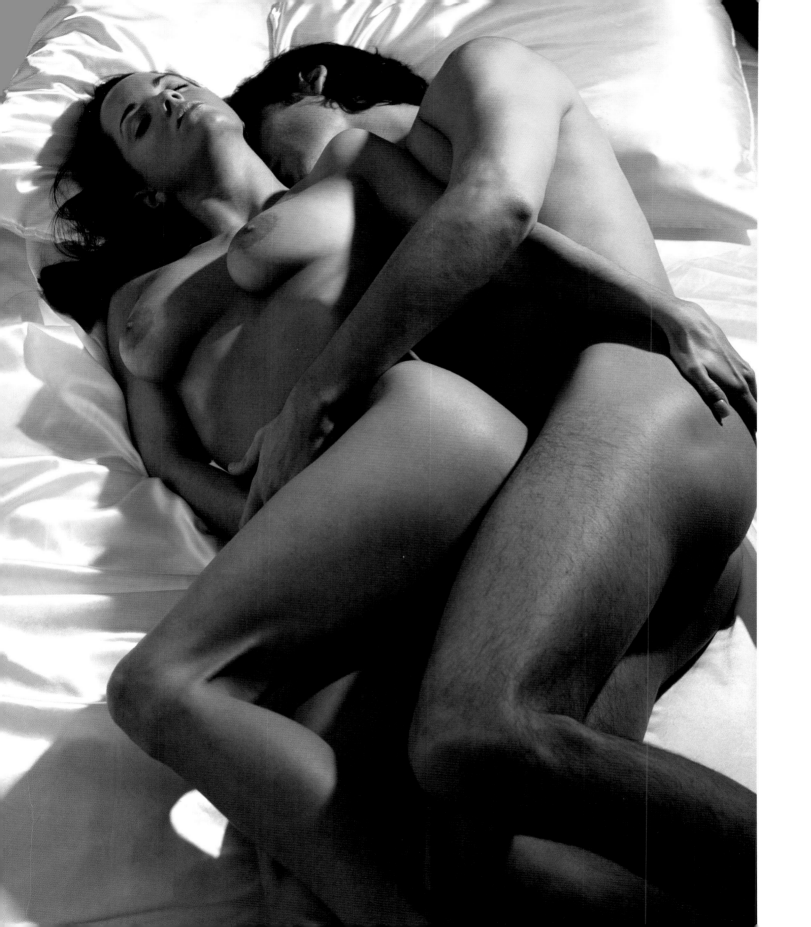

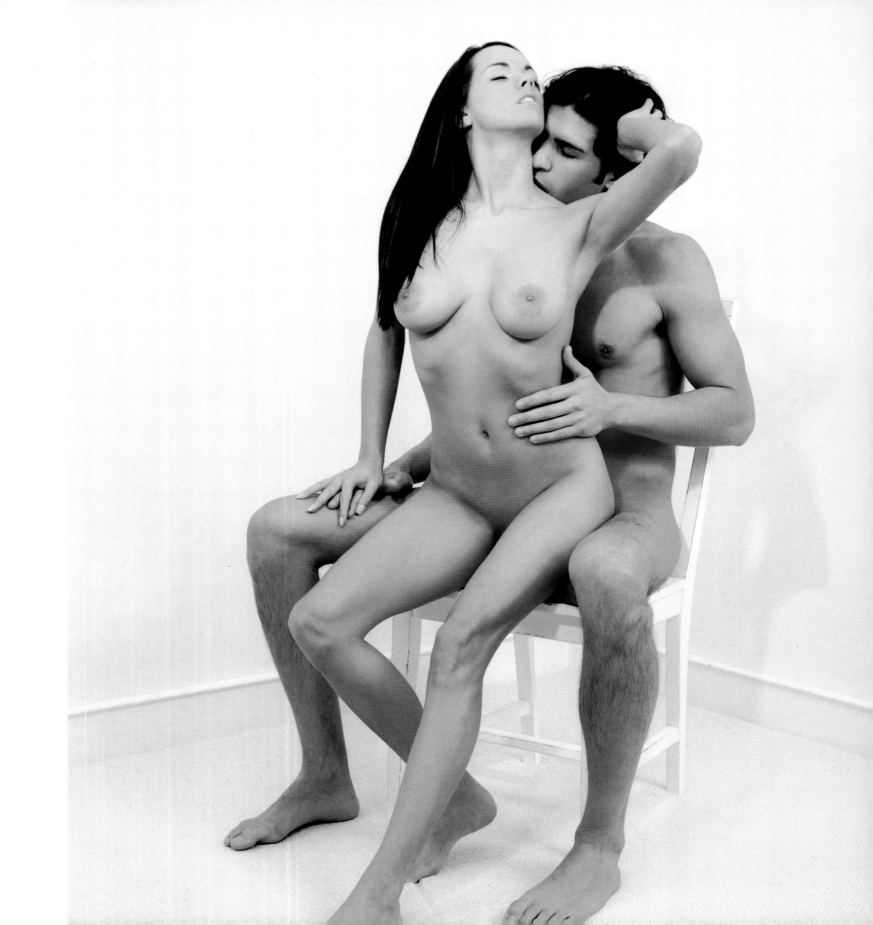

Sitting Position

This is a more versatile position than most people realize. If you think it's just a "nice position" for sexual congress when you're both tired—think again. Penetration can be shallow, but a couple can turn this into a vigorous intercourse position if he grasps her buttocks and she leans back while he thrusts.

BONUS: Climb onto his lap for some intense quickies. Or use the position for good sex for her even without a firm erection for him. She opens her legs and he strokes her clitoris with the underside of his penis.

THE POSITION: He sits in a chair or on the bed with her astride him. She can straddle him face-to-face with her legs brought up to the sides in an overstuffed chair or feet on the floor on either side of a straight-backed chair. Or she can face outward, allowing him more freedom to reach around her body and play with her breasts and clitoris.

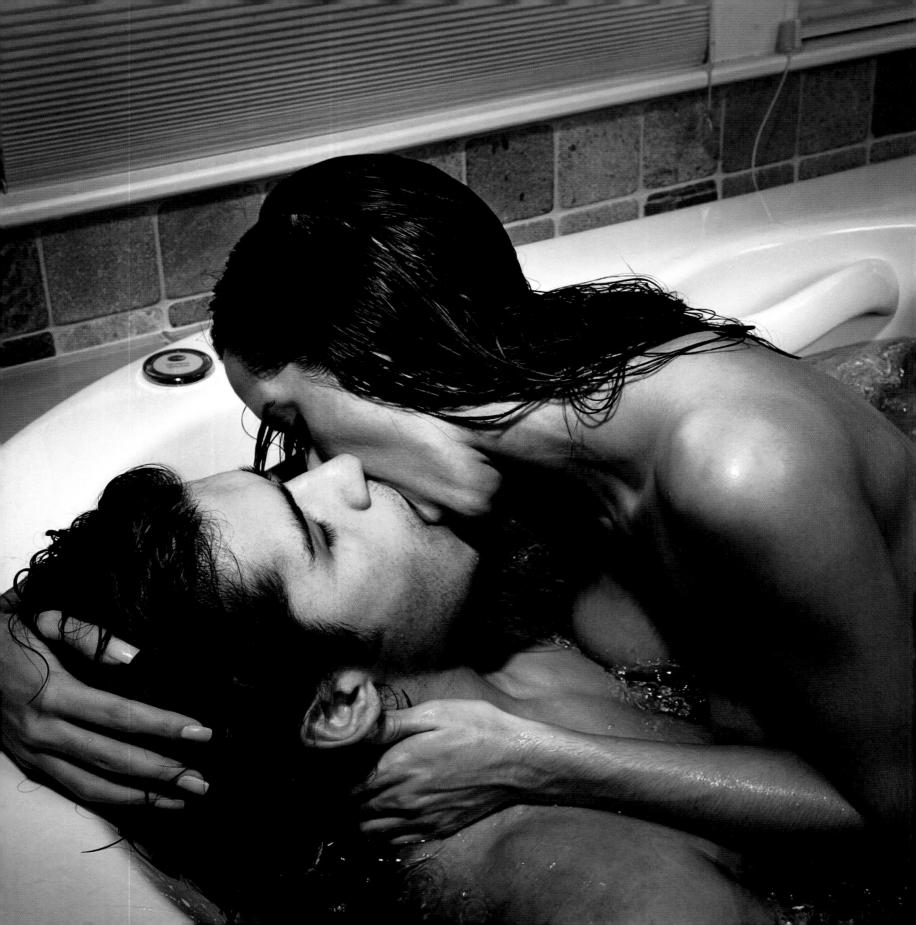

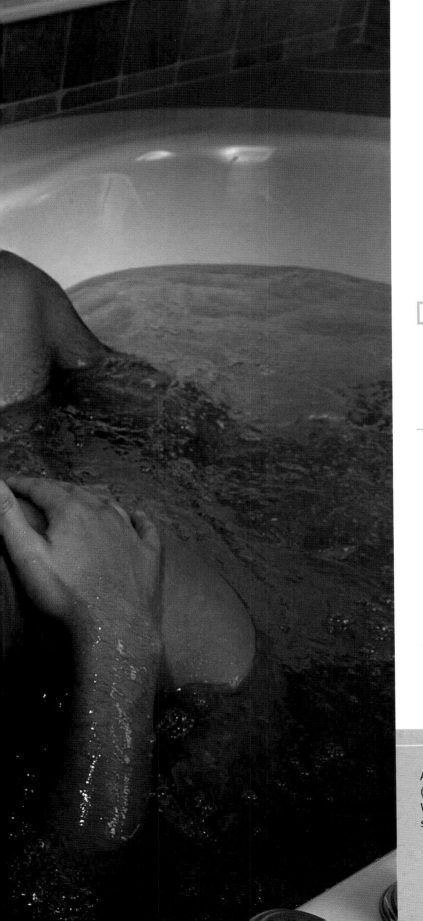

Take it to the river. Okay, the bathtub. Facing the faucet, she kneels in a tub half- filled with warm water. Holding the sides of the tub, she leans forward. He enters from behind. Either of them can use a handheld showerhead to direct water onto her clitoris.

An erotic variation of the female superior position (woman-on-top) is to perform it in a bathtub. Water is a highly sensual playground, and can serve as an exciting alternative to the bedroom.

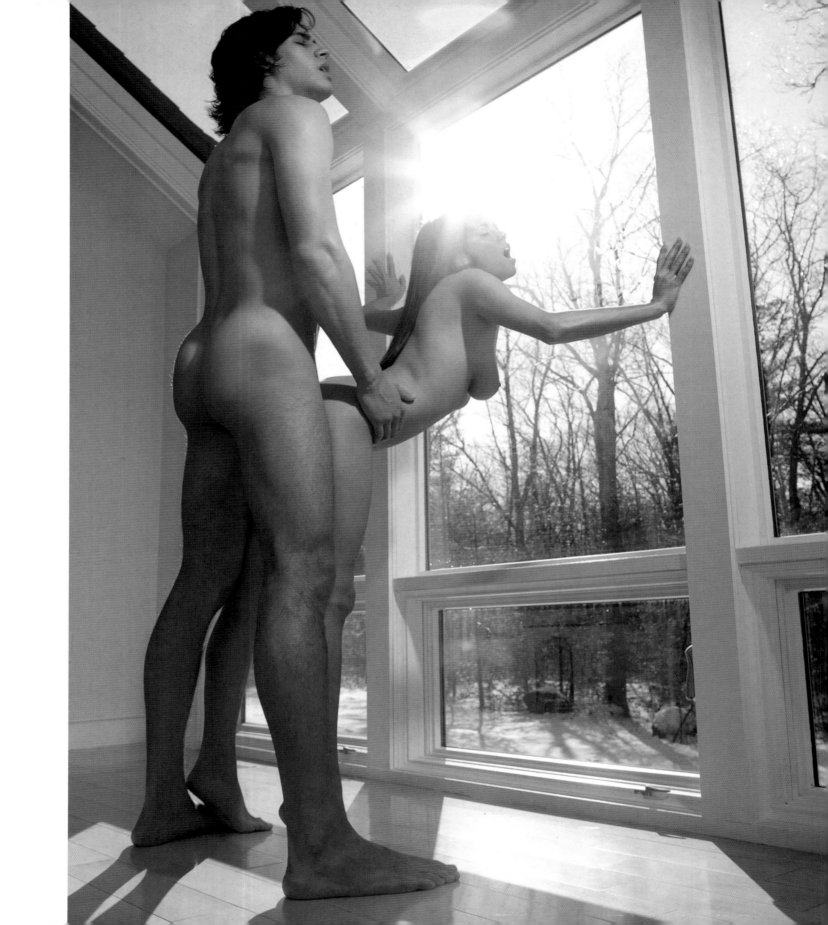

Standing Position

Having intercourse while standing satisfies a need many couples have for dramatic, urgent lovemaking. And it's a great way to begin having sex. You can always slide to the floor and finish in another position.

BONUS: There is no better quickie position.

THE POSITION: He squats slightly while she lowers herself onto him. She wraps one leg around his waist and he holds her buttocks.

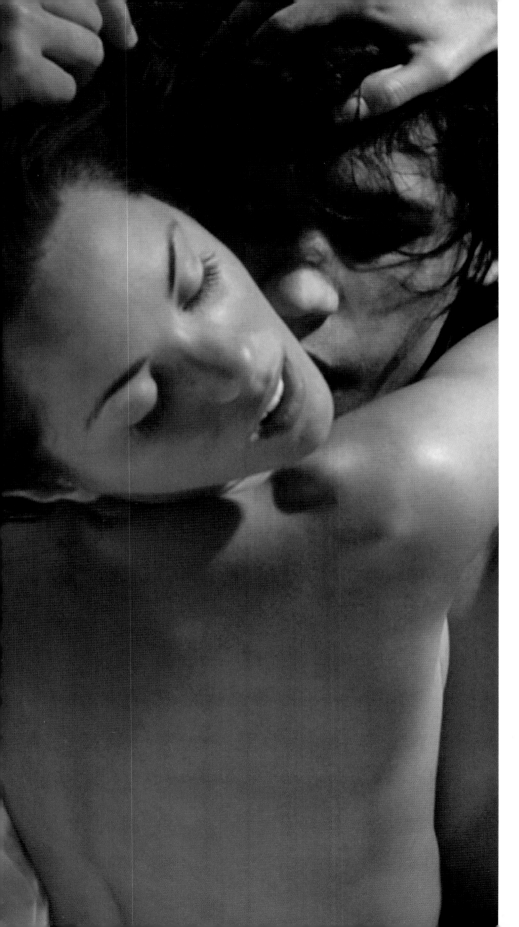

Passion Flower Position

Several years ago the editors of *Redbook* magazine asked me to develop a new sex position for their readers—a position that addressed some common concerns and complaints.

The position had to (1) provide the feeling of greater intimacy for her than the average intercourse position, (2) enable him both to be highly aroused and to sustain intercourse a little longer than he normally could, and (3) give them both exceptional orgasms.

Working with a group of test couples, I developed the Passion Flower, an adaptation of the class Tantric Yab-Yum position (see page 178). The reader response was gratifying. I still teach this position to couples in search of something both hot and intimate.

"Real talk"

"I felt very connected to Jordan in this position," says Caitlin. "And it stimulated my clitoris more than any position we've tried."

And from Jordan: "I couldn't thrust vigorously, so I had to take my time and enjoy the ride. It's like having a built-in delay switch. I could enjoy her arousal and not worry about coming."

Here's how it's done:

Sit in the center of the bed facing each other. Wrap her legs comfortably around his body so that she is sitting on his thighs. His legs can be splayed straight out or bent at the knees—whichever is more comfortable. Each place your right hand at the base of the other's neck and your left hand at the base of the spine. Caress each other's necks. Stroke your lover's back, using upward strokes only. Look into each other's eyes. Kiss with eyes open. Continue kissing and stroking until both are aroused.

Insert his penis into her vagina so that the shaft exerts as much indirect pressure on her clitoris as possible. Rock together, slowly rubbing each other's backs and kissing deeply with eyes open. Because of the intimate clitoral stimulation the position provides, she should be able to reach orgasm this way, while the lack of deep thrusting helps him sustain intercourse without ejaculating.

After her first orgasm, they can move into one of the following variations.

1. HE SITS ON THE BED WITH HIS LEGS WIDE OPEN. She lies back on the bed, facing him, with her body between his legs. He lifts her ankles up against his shoulders and enters her at a comfortable angle. She keeps her thighs closed, creating a tighter grip on his penis. His turn to reach orgasm now—but she can probably have a second one in this position, especially if he stimulates her clitoris.

2. OR SHE LIES ON HER BACK, again between his legs, but with her legs bent at the knees and pulled back against her body until her heels touch her thighs. He sits close to her with his penis opposite her and gently pulls closer until he can comfortably insert his penis.

"It is vitally important to engage in a variety of positions so that sex does not become a boring matter."

— Dr. Ruth Westheimer

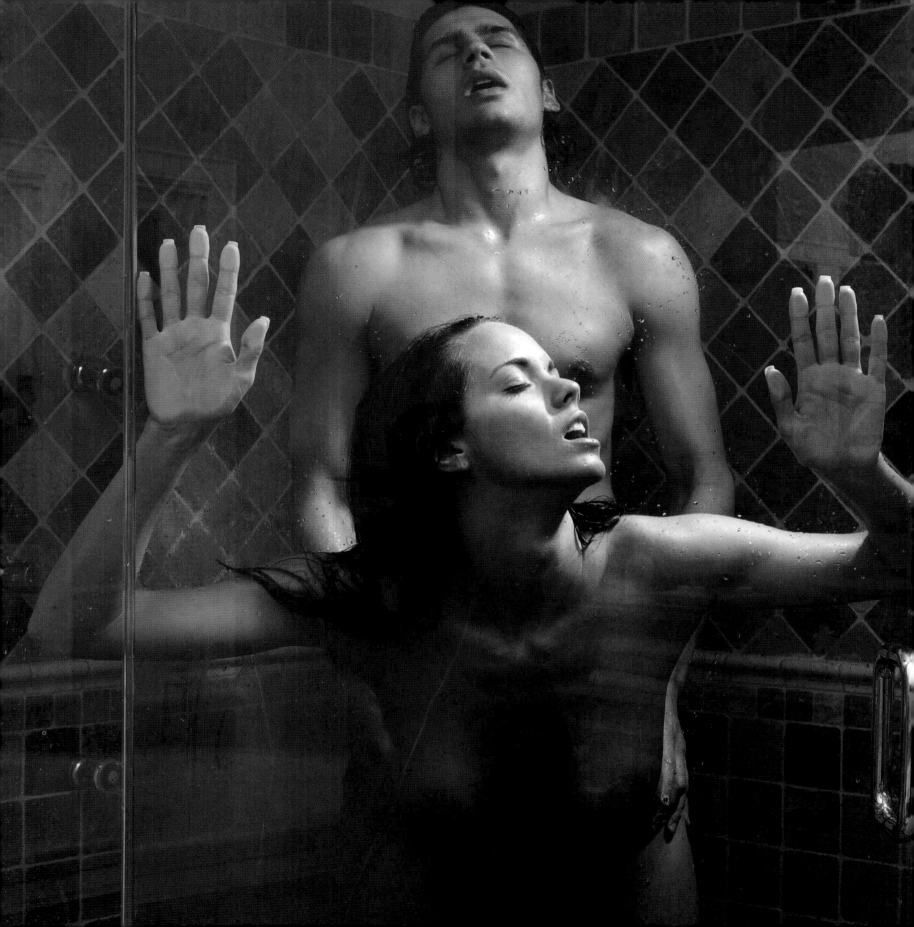

Quickies

Many couples assume that a quickie is something she does occasionally "just for him," because she couldn't possibly come fast enough to make it work for her.

That was your mother's quickie. Today's woman is just as time-pressured, if not more so, than her man. And she can make this position work for her, too.

A few simple techniques for doing that:

- Start on "hot." Because nothing gets you there as quickly as focused self-pleasuring, masturbate (not to orgasm) alone in the bathroom or bedroom before the quickie. In a few minutes, you can bring yourself to his preintercourse level, making a mutual, or nearly so, finish highly likely.

- Masturbate yourself during intercourse.

- Adjust any position to facilitate your hot spot connection. Stand on a little stool, put pillows behind your back or under your ass, make whatever physical adjustments are necessary to get that hot connection immediately.

- Fantasize. Occasionally everyone fantasizes during intercourse. If you have a favorite fantasy that highly arouses you, use it now.

MANUAL STIMULATION DURING INTERCOURSE

More than two-thirds of women don't reach orgasm via intercourse alone.

If you are one of the majority, either you have to touch your clitoris and/or the surrounding tissue during intercourse or he does. One or the other need only insert a finger or two or the side of a hand between your bodies and stroke. If both are too squeamish for manual contact during The Act, then he must arouse you to fever pitch via manual, oral, or a combination of both forms of stimulation before penetration. In that case, you need to be on the verge of orgasm before intercourse.

A little stimulation will trigger release. And you will have that much-desired (and really overvalued) "no hands" orgasm.

A COUPLE'S STORY

Together fifteen years, Peggy and Dick figured out early on that they needed to please each other in bed on a regular basis—at least twice a week, preferably three or four times.

"Otherwise, we fight," she says, laughing mischievously. "We are both strong-willed and opinionated. Sex smooths our rough edges and helps us get along. Without sex, we would always be vying to see who was on top in the relationship."

Here's the surprise inside their story: Their favorite intercourse position is missionary.

"Yes," Peggy says, "I love being masterfully taken by my man. My best orgasms are in the missionary position."

Dick says, "We get very creative with the basic position. Sometimes I am on my knees in front of her, with her legs up on my shoulders or wrapped around my neck. I always make sure that her ass is off the bed so she gets maximum stimulation where she needs it. We go at it hard and fast—but the action is targeted."

Both agree that sex without intercourse isn't as satisfying, even if they both reach orgasm via manual or oral stimulation.

"I love the feeling of penetration," she says. "I need to be penetrated."

No question, he says, that if someday "later on" he needs to take a pill to achieve a good erection, he will do that.

"Intercourse is the core sexual activity for a couple," Dick says. "Whenever I read something in one of her magazines about men and women placing 'too much emphasis' on intercourse, I think, They don't know how to do it right or they wouldn't say that."

"Intercourse in the man on top position is the most intensely pleasurable experience a woman can have," Peggy says.

Every couple should have a no-fail intercourse position.

What is that?

The one that leads assuredly to orgasm nearly every time—for both lovers—in fifteen minutes or less. That makes it a bit longer than a quickie, somewhat shorter than they might like to make love if they had more time—but just right for keeping a busy couple sexually connected and satisfied. Whether their fail-safe position is missionary, woman on top, rear entry, or another doesn't make a difference; as long as it works for them most of the time, it works perfectly.

You've heard this before, but the keys to success are twofold: strong PC muscles (see page 36) and her ability to have an orgasm whenever she wants one. (See the "Orgasm Loop," page 149.)

Perfect your technique in your favorite position and you will have a no-fail intercourse position, too.

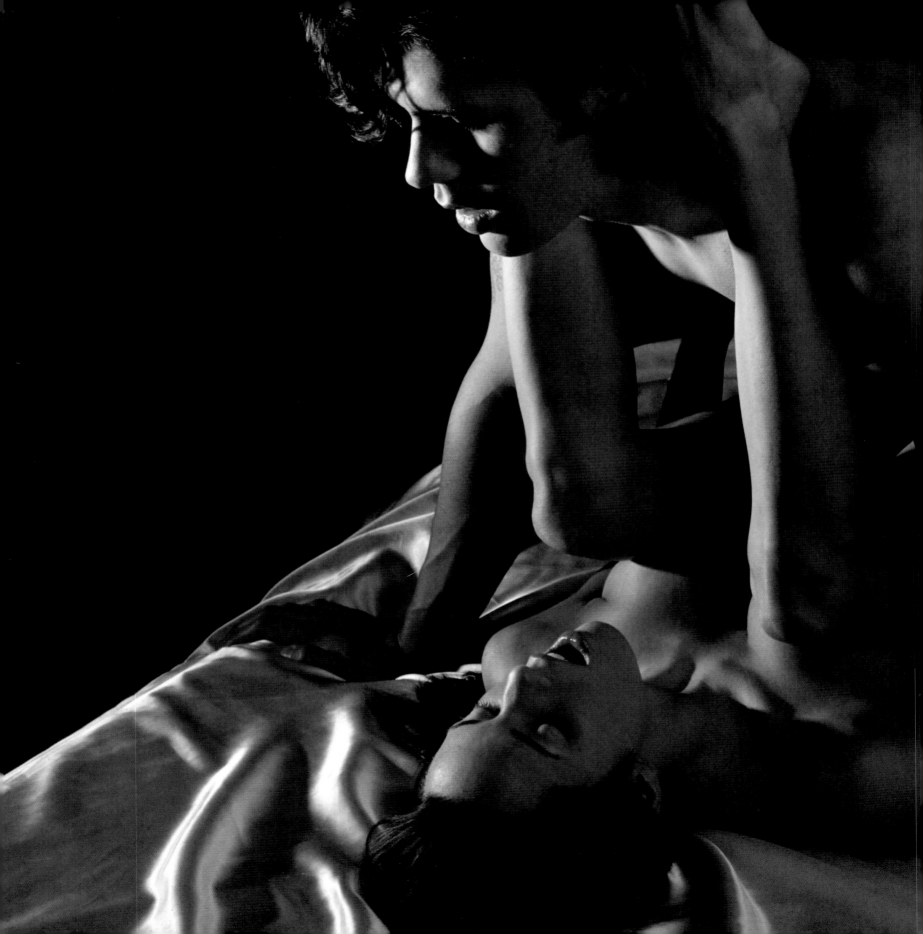

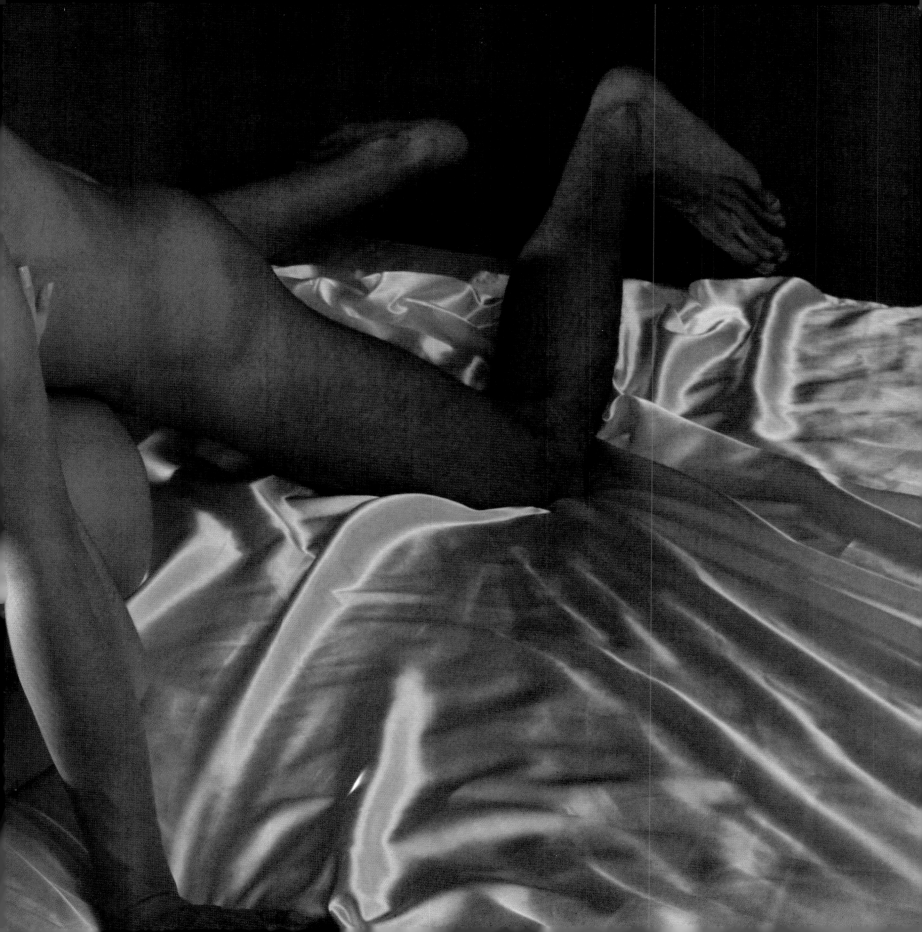

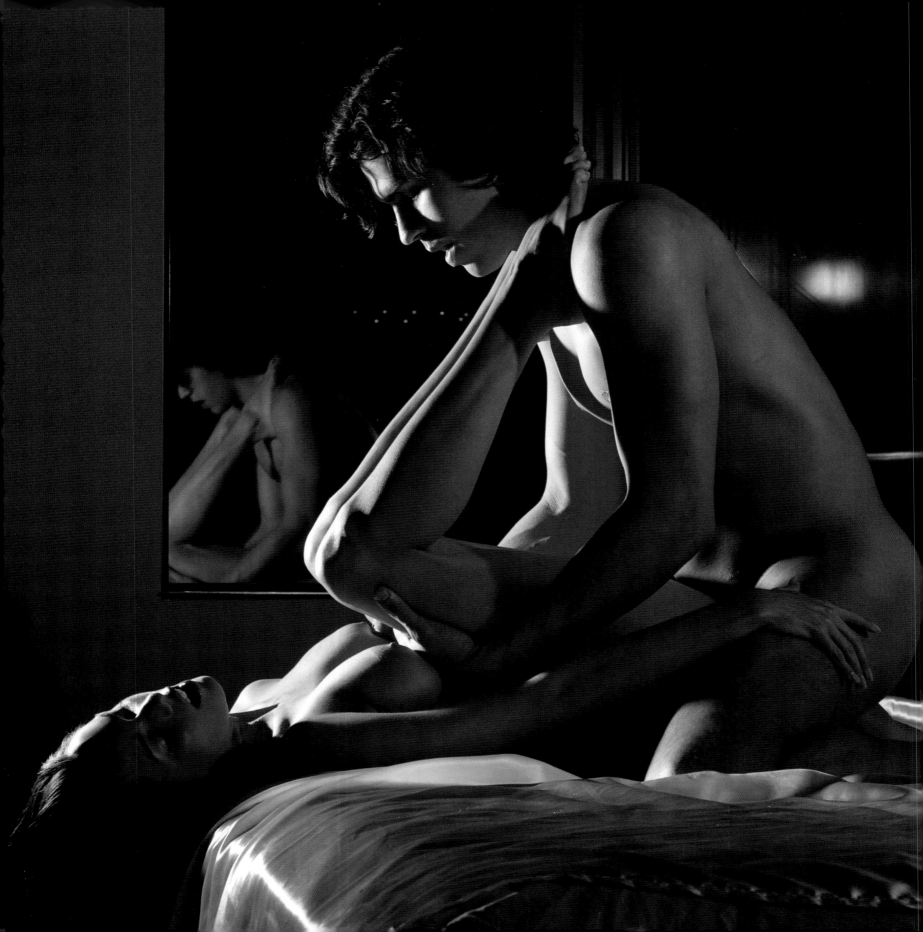

Hot Spot Intercourse

Connect your hot spots with your lover's during intercourse—and you increase the likelihood she will reach orgasm. And you will both experience a higher level of arousal and bigger orgasms. Yes, the hot spots are that important.

Make whatever adjustments to intercourse positions are necessary to bring your hot spots into alignment. Her clitoris, AFE Zone, and G-spot need to interact with the head of his penis, his frenulum, and his raphe.

In the missionary position, put her feet on his shoulders, or pull her knees up to her chest and place her feet flat against his chest. Or have him support her legs with his forearms under her knees.

In the female superior position, she should lean either back or forward (rather than sitting straight up).

In the spoon position, she lies on her side with her back toward him, bent slightly at the knees and waist. Also bent slightly at the knees and waist, he enters her from behind.

Technique Tip

THE EXCELLENT HOT SPOT CONNECTION POSITION

I adapted the X from the Kama Sutra position "woman acting the part of man."

It may sound like an awkward position as you're reading the directions, but it is really very comfortable, even for overweight people.

Imagine that your bodies form an X with the connection at the genitals. He sits at the edge of the bed with his back straight, one leg outstretched on the bed and the other outstretched toward the floor. Or, if he prefers, he can brace that leg against a straight-backed chair placed near the bed. Her back supported by pillows, she sits astride her lover with both legs braced on his shoulders.

You won't fall right into this position the first time you try it. But you will the second or third time around. The hot spot connection is so good that it's definitely worth the trouble.

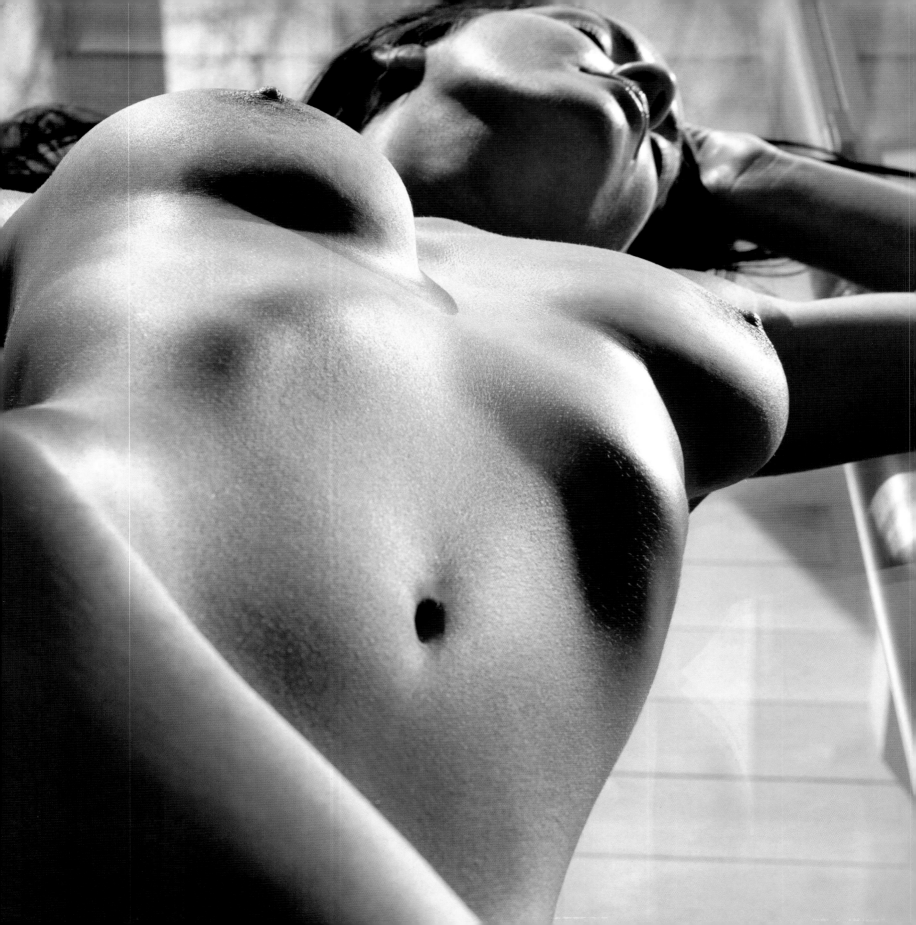

Changing Positions

How often should you change positions during intercourse?

Change positions when you need to change the genital stimulation. He may need to pull back to keep from ejaculating too soon—or get into a position where he can thrust harder so he can ejaculate. She may need to have repeated stimulation to reach orgasm and so he needs to stay in place to keep giving her what she needs.

Don't change positions just to impress your partner with your physical dexterity. On the other hand, don't stay in one place so long you are getting muscle cramps. There has to be a middle ground.

Sometimes it's good to change positions because your intimacy needs to fluctuate during lovemaking. Maybe you want to move from driving hard in the rear entry position to a face-to-face position so you can look into each other's eyes. Let your partner know when you need a change by shifting your body slightly or whispering, "I want you this way now."

Intercourse with Other Body Parts

Every now and then a man can be satisfied by having intercourse with a part of your body that has no orifice. If you're not exactly in the mood but want to do something for him, or just something different, this works.

Men adore women's breasts. Making love to breasts is "intramammary intercourse"—or lovemaking *de l'espagnol*. In the days before reliable birth control, Spanish men attempted to convince their women that this was a safe and satisfying substitute for intercourse. Well, for them, it was.

Here's how it works:

He holds your breasts together around his penis and gently thrusts. The sensations are exciting for both, especially if you have very sensitive breasts. When he's ready to ejaculate, if he holds his penis and directs his ejaculate so that he is forming "pearls" around your throat, you're doing String of Pearls, highly touted in Internet sex chat rooms. (Quite possibly that variation occurred to our Spanish ancestors, too. Every generation and culture reinvents. We never truly invent anything.)

Your armpits, buttocks, and inner thighs can also be used as alternative areas for intercourse. In some societies—not Christian ones—these ways of having intercourse were not only sanctioned but encouraged as ways of preventing unwanted pregnancy. The Zulu warriors, for example, were permitted to move their penises between the thighs of virgins as long as they didn't enter a vagina. The practice was called "wiping of the spears."

Men always love to watch their penis in action. Women haven't had much opportunity to watch—except in porn films. You might find this practice very exciting for that reason alone.

Anal Intercourse

Heterosexual anal intercourse is much more commonly practiced now than it was even a decade ago. For example, ten years ago 11 percent of *Cosmopolitan* readers had experienced anal sex—and now 39 percent have.

Some women balk. Some women tolerate it, especially for the right guy. Some women love it.

With the right man in the right moment, anal intercourse is an incomparable erotic experience. Like caviar and anchovies, it isn't an everyday thing. This is special sex with a special man.

Anal Intercourse

- Sex play should include cunnilingus and manual stimulation of her clitoris. The goal: intense arousal before you go near her anus.

- She assumes a comfortable position. For many women the rear entry position with chest flat on the bed and ass elevated is the best position. There are other options. For example, she can lie on her back with legs straight up or ankles resting on his shoulders while he kneels between her legs and enters her.

- Always use a specially designed anal condom and *plenty* of a lubricant. (The anus, unlike the vagina, is not self-lubricating.) The condom is essential to keep bacteria out of your urethra. Using a finger protected by a disposable "finger cot," insert copious amounts of lube into her anus.

- Start very slowly.

- As you press the head of your penis against her anus, encourage her to relax the sphincter muscles in her rectum.

- Don't force your penis inside her. Ask her to bear down on the head of your penis until you are past the sphincter muscles.

- Following her lead, thrust slowly and carefully. Let her control the depth of penetration and the speed of thrusting.

- While you are thrusting, either you or she should be stimulating her clitoris.

- With any luck, she will reach orgasm.

- Afterward, don't insert your penis into her vagina until you have removed the condom and thoroughly washed your penis and hands. You both risk contracting a urinary tract infection if the cleanliness rules are not scrupulously followed.

"My ass is my very own back door to heaven.

As he enters me, I let go of the tensing. . . .

I am addicted to extreme physical endurance."

— Toni Bentley,
author of *The Surrender:
An Erotic Memoir*
about her obsession with anal sex

A COUPLE'S STORY

Beth resisted. Jack persisted. How many anal sex stories begin this way?

"Most of the women I knew who had tried it said they hated it," Beth says. "They said it hurt. The only women who seemed to like anal sex were in the letters to Penthouse Forum, not exactly a reliable source. I really did not want to go there."

She asked Jack, "Why? Why do you want my ass so much?"

He had all the usual answers: "I want your ass because it's so beautiful, because no one else has had it, because I want to be inside your tight, hot, most private place."

Finally, she was moved by the strength of his desire. Or, as he remembers it: He wore her down.

"I was scared," she remembers. "He promised to take it slow and stop if I couldn't take it. We used a lot of lube when the time came. But the most important part: He got me so hot through extended foreplay that I was almost ready for anal sex."

Jack says, "I kissed her long and slow the way she loves. Then I kissed my way down her body. I put the flat of my hand between her wet lips while I nibbled on her inner thighs. By the time I got to her clitoris, she was hot."

He pulled away before her orgasm. Feeling "erotic dread, wanting and fearing," in the pit of her stomach, she "assumed the position," a lower, more accessible version of rear entry. He took his time circling her anus with lubricated fingers, inserting first one, then two, covered in heavy dollops of lube.

"I gasped when I felt his head push into me," she says. "Yes, it hurt . . . but it hurt good. I wanted him inside me. I pushed back against him, encouraging him. His penis felt huge and hard, but I wanted it."

Beth stroked her clitoris with one hand as Jack moved slowly and rhythmically in and out, going a little deeper each time. She was panting and sweating. "Don't stop," she told him.

"I took all of him inside me on my very first time, and came in a different way than I ever had before," she says.

"It was an extremely erotic experience that we enjoy re-creating when we're both in the mood for something a little different from our normal sex routine," Jack says.

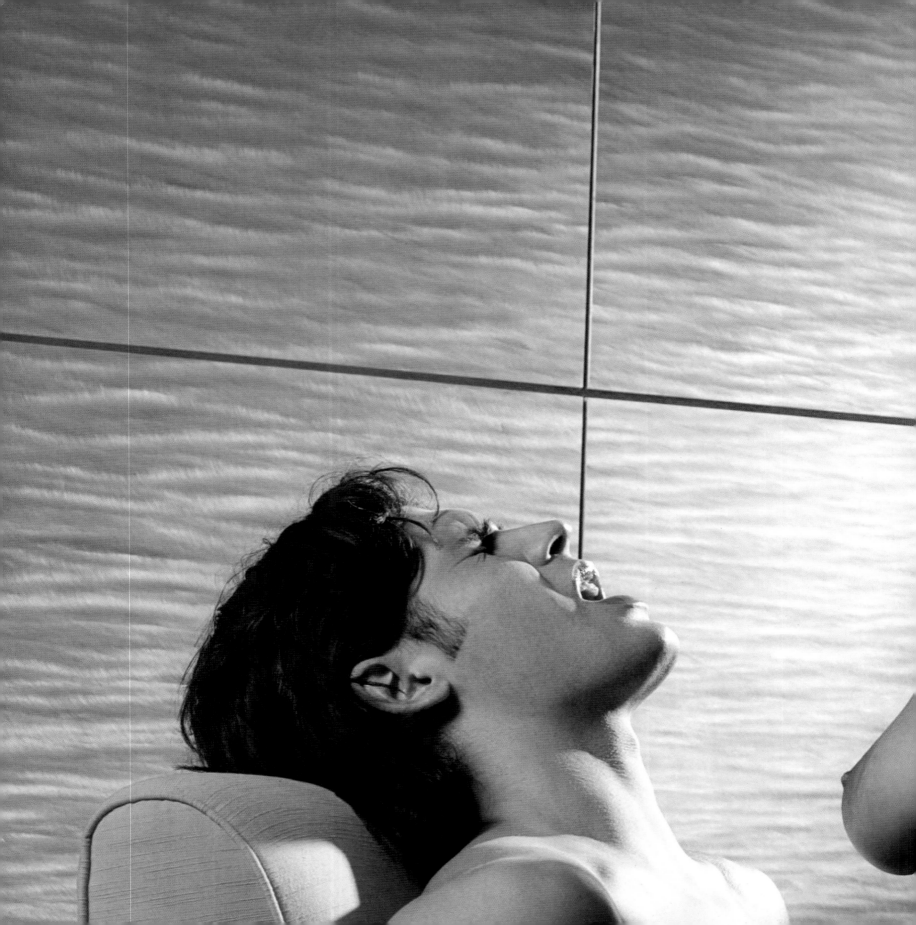

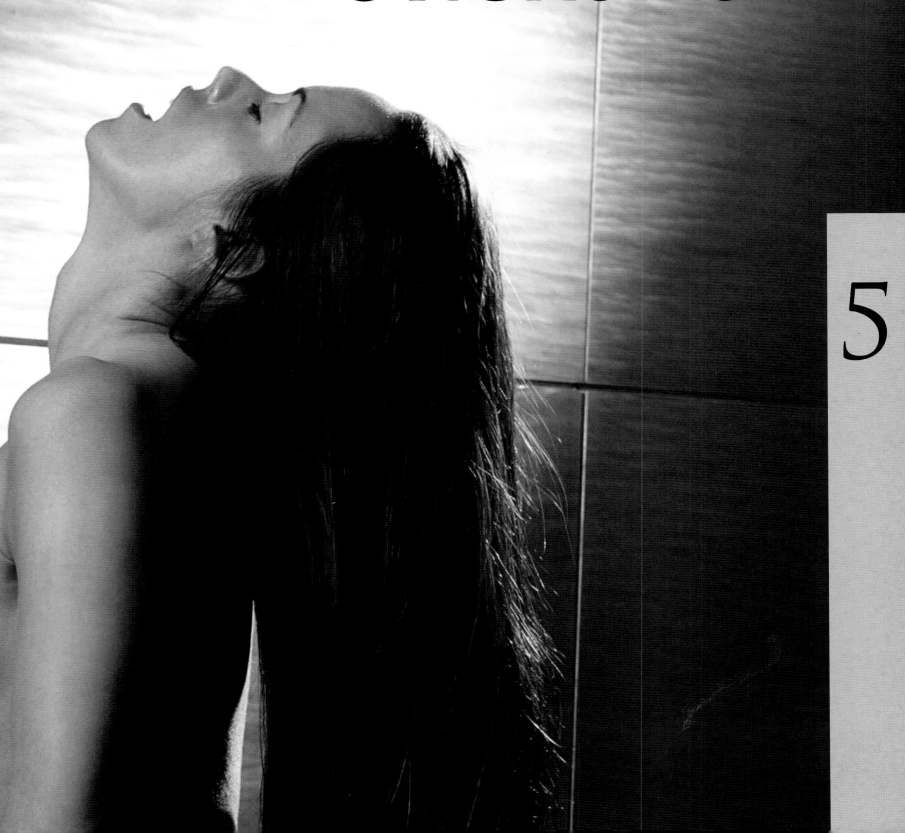

ORGASMS

5

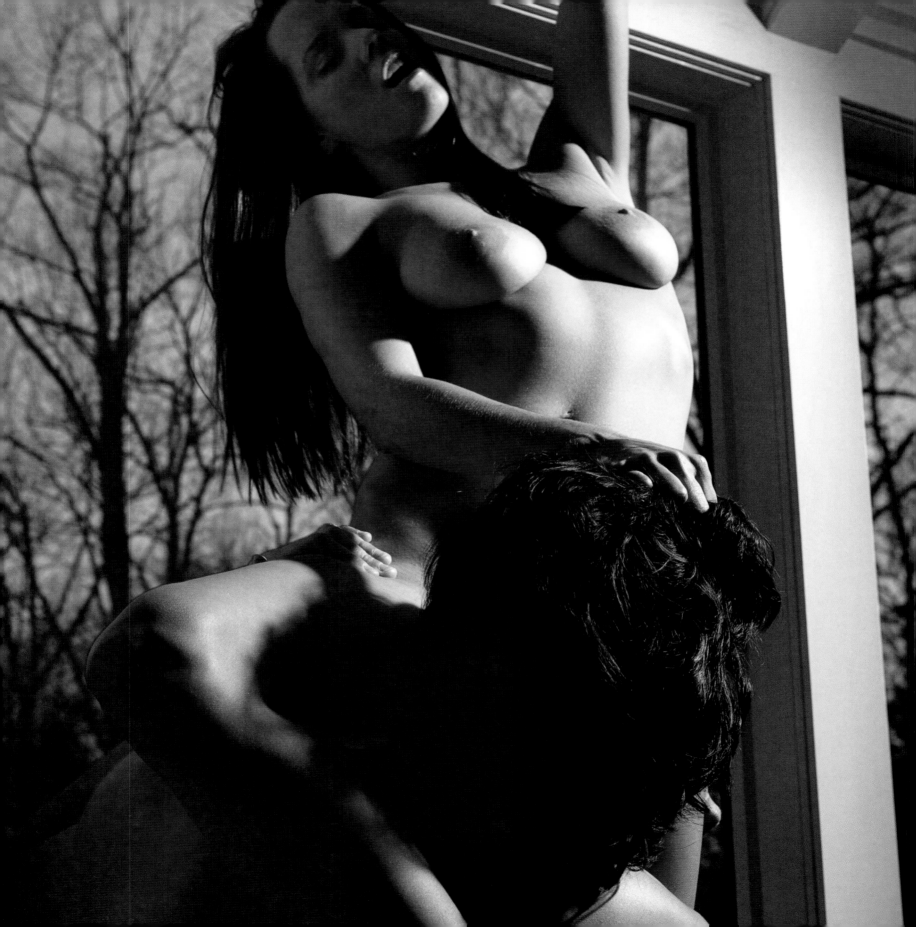

THE GLORY OF ORGASMS

"Electric flesh arrows transverse the body.

A rainbow of color strikes the eyelid. . . .

It is the glory of orgasm."

— Anaïs Nin,
Erotic writer, from her journals

Glorious whole-body event or another tepid night in bed when you act to convince him that it was all that?

Which describes orgasm for most women? For you?

The word comes from the Greek *orgao*, meaning to be full of passion and pleasure. Orgasms vary from man to man, woman to woman, and individually from time to time. They are sometimes thrilling and intense, sometimes mild, diffuse, pleasurable but subtle.

Ironically, male and female orgasms are more alike than different. Each gender experiences orgasm as a series of rhythmic contractions that release the tension built up by sexual arousal. Yet his orgasm is almost biologically inevitable, while hers is problematic. He will come, she—maybe not. Some experts put that difference down to evolution: He had to reach orgasm/ejaculation to propagate the race; she had only to receive his sperm. *But*, because his orgasm is connected to ejaculation and thus limited by his refractory period and she has no similar restriction, she really has the potential to experience the multiple, extended, and otherwise amazing orgasms that will likely elude him.

Orgasms! They are sublime, they are disappointing, they are reliable, they are serendipitous. They are all these things and more. We obsess over them. Look up "orgasm" online and you will get millions of hits, more responses than you can read. Women do not feel like real women if they can't reach orgasm. Men measure themselves as lovers in the numbers of orgasms they "give" their partners.

What we believe about orgasm—largely but not entirely *female* orgasm—has been linked more to the religious, social, and political climate of the times—and geography—than to scientific research. The idea that women deserve to have an orgasm is a fairly modern one, born in the twentieth century in the West. They did, however, have it figured out in India five thousand years ago, when sexuality was sacred and the vagina (yoni) was worshipped along with the penis (lingam). That men should give their lovers the first orgasm via cunnilingus is the lasting legacy of the baby boom generation.

In more recent years, the power and possibility of *orgasm* has been hyped beyond actual or potential reality. Books about extended orgasm promise more in the title than they deliver on the page. *The One Hour Orgasm*, for example, guarantees that hour of pleasure by redefining orgasm. According to this new definition, "Orgasm begins when the genital area is feeling better than any other part of the body."

Orgasm! It is good. It can be as possible for women as for men. We don't have to hype it any more than we should confine it inside religious, social, or political boundary lines. And you can take this good thing and make it better, even best.

What Orgasm Is

HER ORGASM

When a woman is aroused, blood flow increases to the vagina, causing lubrication and swelling her inner and outer lips and her clitoris. With enough intense physical and psychological stimulation, she will reach orgasm. The vagina, sphincter, and uterus contract simultaneously. The blood congealed in her vaginal area suddenly rushes back to the rest of her body.

The entire explosion, or set of contractions, generally lasts three to twenty seconds, with intervals of less than a second between the first three to six contractions. Some women experience single orgasms lasting a minute or more. Some women feel postorgasmic contractions up to twenty-four hours later. And some women do feel the orgasm radiating throughout their bodies.

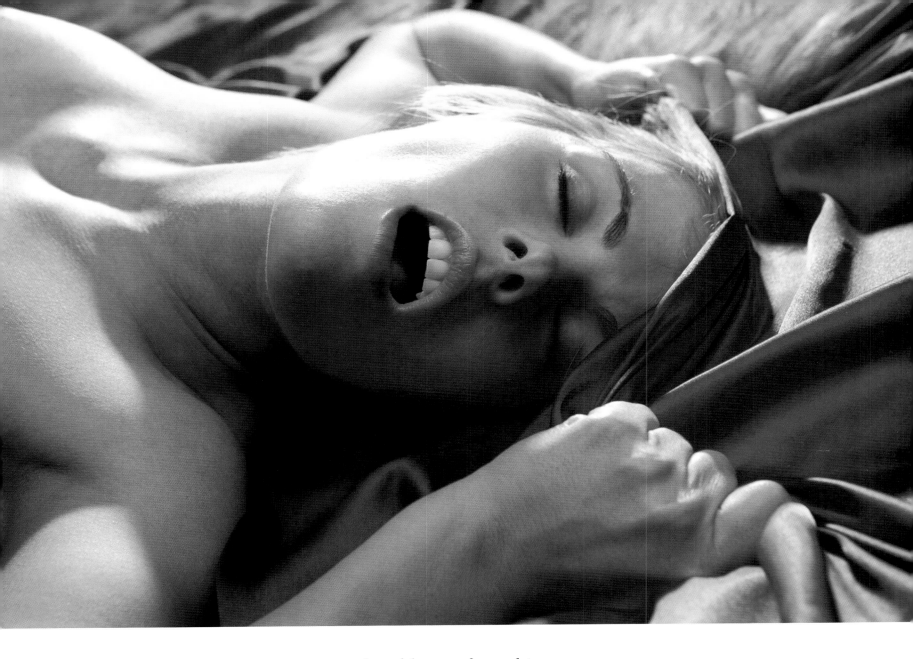

"*Ten seconds of heavy breathing,*

roll your head from side to side, simulate

a slight asthma attack, and die a little."

— Actress Candice Bergen
(on how to fake an orgasm on-screen or off)

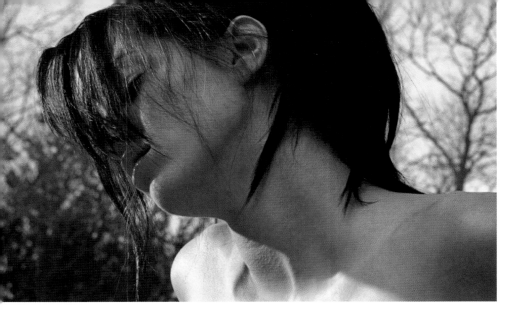

"Is faking orgasm an

antifeminist act? I don't know.

"A recent study showed that

a woman's brain waves can tell you

if she has actually had an orgasm

—or faked one.

"So whatever you do, don't get

involved with a neurologist."

— Maureen Dowd
Columnist for *The New York
Times* and author of
Are Men Necessary?
in a nerve.com interview

Clitoral or vaginal orgasm?

The debate continues. Sigmund Freud distinguished clitoral from vaginal orgasm and labeled the former "immature" and "neurotic." The adolescent girl experienced clitoral orgasm during masturbation, he reasoned. Once she became sexually active with a partner, she switched to vaginal orgasms—or so Freud thought. The man didn't know much about female anatomy.

In 1953 Alfred Kinsey, Ph.D., in his landmark study *Sexual Behavior in the Human Female*, said all female orgasms were achieved by clitoral stimulation, either direct or indirect. His findings were endorsed a decade later by pioneer sex researchers William Masters, M.D., and Virginia Johnson, Ph.D., who isolated the orgasm in a lab setting and measured and quantified the results as women writhed in pleasure on the sterile tables. The clitoral orgasm theory became the prevailing opinion among sexologists until 1980, when Beverly Whipple and John Perry claimed their research proved the existence of the G-spot and therefore put the orgasm back inside the vagina—at least sometimes.

A few years later, Helen Singer Kaplan, Ph.D., a pioneer in the field of sex therapy and founder of the country's first clinic for sexual disorders, insisted that 75 percent of women do not reach orgasm during intercourse without some kind of directly clitoral stimulation. A host of studies over the years have supported her theory.

Vaginal or clitoral?

Almost every woman can have a clitoral orgasm. Some women can have a vaginal orgasm. And no orgasm is politically incorrect. Enjoy whatever you can get.

Why do women fake orgasm?

To end the sex!

Yes, women fake so he will stop now.

"End the sex" is the primary reason for faking, which women have been giving for the past two decades. And the numbers of women who report faking orgasms in surveys hasn't changed, either. In 1994 Shere Hite wrote in *The Hite Report* that half the women who responded to her survey said they faked orgasm. A recent *Glamour* magazine poll reported the same number. These are conservative numbers.

Most women have faked at least once or twice in their sex lives. And, as Sally told Harry in the classic film *When Harry Met Sally*, most men don't believe women have been faking with them. (Remember when Elaine told Jerry on the hit sitcom *Seinfeld* that she had been faking with him? He was stunned.)

Faking is, of course, counterproductive. In faking that orgasm, she's telling him: Yes, what you just did worked—keep doing it.

THE TOP FIVE REASONS WOMEN FAKE ORGASMS

To end the sex. She's tired, it's not happening, she has other things to do. He won't quit until she says, "Yes, yes, oh, yes!" (She can't say, "No, no, oh, no!" and get out of it nicely, can she?)

She is too stressed, tired, "not in the mood" to have an orgasm, but she doesn't want to hurt his feelings. She does the "polite" thing and says with her prettily faked orgasm, "I had a wonderful time; thank you very much." It's a new relationship and she's feeling shy. She doesn't know how to show and tell him what she wants. And she's a little embarrassed to let go in front of him, anyway.

She doesn't want him to ask, "What's wrong?" Then she has to say, "But I love sex even when I don't come." If he believes her, he may stop trying so hard. And if he doesn't believe her, he feels hurt and rejected. Anyway, that's what she thinks.

She thinks she is expected to come. Porn stars always do, don't they?

How you can stop faking

STEP ONE: Acknowledge that men don't "give" women orgasms. No matter how good a lover he is, he can't make you come. You give yourself up to the pleasure of sex or you won't have an orgasm, no matter what he does.

Ideally, he and she should acknowledge this universal truth and take the performance pressure off him. Realistically, she had better acknowledge it to herself if she wants more real orgasms than faked ones. The Big Talk about the meaning of orgasms isn't necessary if she can accept the internal message.

STEP TWO: The more you worry about having an orgasm and the harder you "try" to have one, the more difficult reaching orgasm becomes. You've heard this one before: Relax. But you have to figure out how to do it.

STEP THREE: Be an active sex partner. Show him what you want by guiding his mouth and hands where you need them to go. Tell him what you want—but don't make it sound like you're reading prepared lecture notes. When you give a man instructions in bed, make them sound like breathless requests. You're begging for it. He loves that.

Can't pull off the begging, you say? Sure you can. It requires the same acting skills as faking an orgasm.

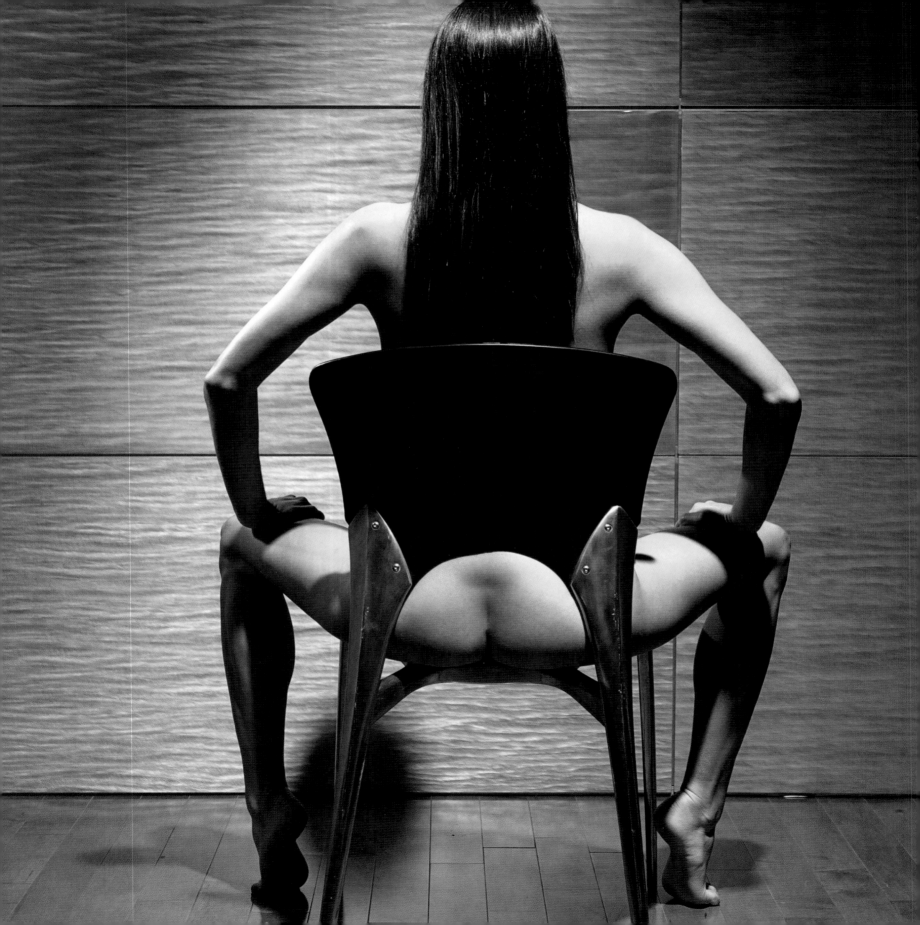

A WOMAN'S STORY

I am a desirable and sexy woman—according to the men I've known. And I was a lingerie model for three years back in the late 80s. If you strip to bits of silk and lace and pose, you're easy about sex, right?

For years I faked more orgasms than I had. I got better at faking as I had a few more of the real ones. Faking is like any kind of acting. You do better at it if you have some experience with the real thing, whether it's sadness or orgasm. I could get so carried away with making noise and thrashing around that I almost believed myself.

I know all the reasons not to fake. It doesn't help my partner give me a real orgasm. Lying isn't nice. And faking is not an intimate act. If you fake, you don't get close to your partner. The afterplay cuddling is a lie. But I was okay with that, because I like keeping my distance most of the time.

Having an orgasm with a man is letting go. The truth is: I sometimes don't want to have one with a man because I don't want to give him that or to lose myself with him. When I was married, I had a lot of orgasms with him in the beginning. When things started going wrong, I didn't want to have them with him. So I faked.

I never had a problem reaching orgasm via masturbation. Sex and orgasm are separate things. Having one can be a lot of work if you aren't into the guy and into the moment.

Lately I've been happy and content with a man. He knows the difference between a real orgasm and a faked one. I can't fool him with the fake. He does things to my clit with his fingers and tongue that may not be any different from what other men have done. But it all feels different.

We talk about sex. He tells me about his past, about the other women—and it doesn't make me crazy. It's all interesting to me. Sometimes it's sexy.

The second time we made love, he asked me if I didn't come with men and I said, I don't care if I come; it doesn't matter. He tied my wrists to his bed and went down on me until I came and came. His face was slick with sweat and my juices when he finally came up for air. He kissed me hard and said, "Taste yourself; that's the truth; don't ever lie to me again."

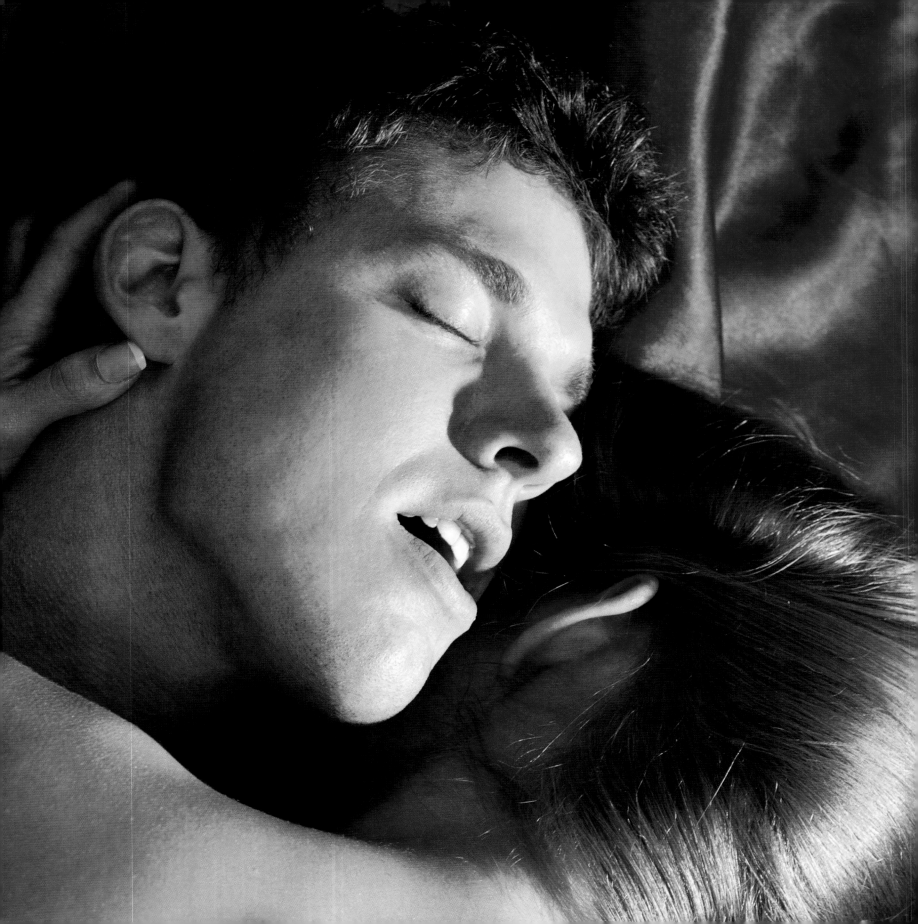

Spiking Her Orgasm

What can you do to make her orgasm more special, intense, memorable?

These little moves make a big difference:

If she has sensitive nipples, pinch them as she comes.

Kiss her with your eyes wide open as she's coming. It's a tender yet passionate act—and shows her that you are not afraid of being very intimate with her.

Whisper terms of endearment. Instead of "Yeah, baby, give it to me," say, "You're so beautiful," "You feel so good," and even "I love you," if you do.

If you are giving her an orgasm via cunnilingus, stimulate her G-spot at the same time. Her orgasm will feel as if it's coming from both places—and will reverberate through her vagina.

HIS ORGASM

According to the prevailing opinion of Western sex therapists, male orgasm and ejaculation are the same thing. Some sexologists, however, share the Eastern belief that male orgasm, like female, is a psychophysical experience that typically includes ejaculation, but not always. These "experts" separate the pleasure of the rhythmic contractions from the expulsion of semen. (See "His Male Multiples," page 156.)

However you define his orgasm—with ejaculation or not—arousal leads to the engorgement of blood vessels. During orgasm, the blood rushes back into his body. He experiences contractions of his penis and surrounding genital area as pleasurable sensations similar in timing sequence and length to her orgasm.

Unless he has figured out how to have those nonejaculatory orgasms, he needs a refractory period following orgasm before he can get another erection and have another orgasm. In young men, the refractory period may be a matter of minutes. In older men, it can be twenty-four hours or more.

Spiking his orgasm

What can you do to make his orgasm more special, intense, memorable?

Two subtle but effective moves:

Pinch or bite his nipple at the moment of orgasm.

Make a dramatic pause. If he's on top, grab his buttocks at the moment of orgasm, use your PC muscle to pull him in a little deeper. Make eye contact with him at the same time.

A major part of the satisfaction men get from sex is the ego boost that results from also making their partners climax.

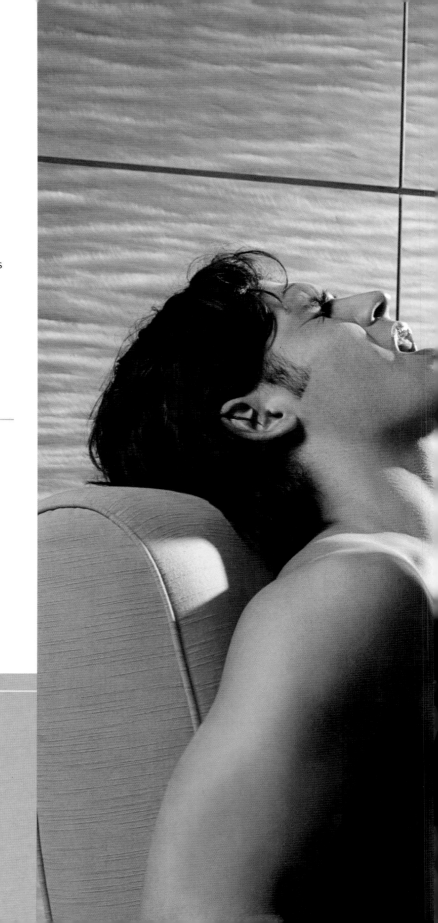

THE HIP ROCK 'N' ROLL

If he's on top and close to orgasm, grab his hip bones
or buttocks and rock him, side to side or back and forth.
When you control the direction of his pelvic movements,
you also control the speed of thrusting and the depth
of penetration. To him, it feels as if you are pulling the
orgasm out of him in a very explosive way.

If you're on top and he's close to orgasm, put your hands
on his hips and pull him toward you. Keep your body
weight on your knees so that you aren't bearing down
on his hips. Again, he will feel as if you're pulling that
orgasm out of him.

And if you want to give him something really special,
fellate him to orgasm. When he's near ejaculation,
take his pelvis in both hands and rock him toward you
so that he goes deeper into your mouth. And swallow.

When a woman is on top, and the man is
close to orgasm, try to extend his physical
and mental build-up by temporarily stopping
movement. This brief cooling-off period will
enable you both to simultaneously ascend
to climax again.

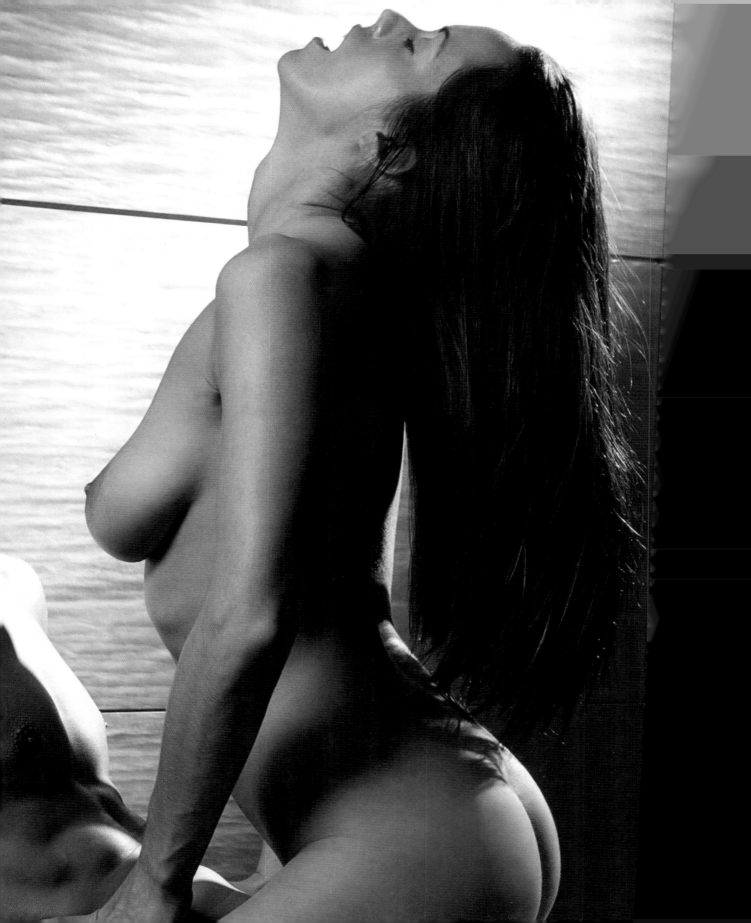

The Butterfly Quiver

Any woman can feel like a sex goddess if she perfects this move. It couldn't be easier. Simply flex your PC muscle in time with his thrusting. When his erection is very hard, have him slow down and let you control the thrusting dynamics of intercourse.

His cooperation is important. The Butterfly Quiver is most effective when he doesn't thrust vigorously. For greater control, shift to the female superior position if you aren't there already.

Now flex your PC muscle in a continuous pattern of tightening (as you pull him inside) and releasing (as you push him out), replicating the pattern of a butterfly's pulsating wings. Make the butterfly flutter as fast as you can as he nears ejaculation.

When you have developed a strong PC muscle, you can make him feel as if the ejaculate is being pulled from his body, a thrill for both of you. Both of your orgasms will be intense, often multiple—and amazing.

Delaying his orgasm

Men often lament that they reached orgasm "too soon." That usually means they wanted the sex to last longer because they disappointed their lover. She probably agrees with him. He may have given her an orgasm via cunnilingus or she may have had one manually. They both want the period of thrusting to last longer.

This is the male/female sexual equation reduced to its most basic element: Men want to penetrate—and women want to be penetrated. If you love a woman, you want to be inside her—and for more than just a few minutes. If you love a man, you want to feel him inside you—and, again, for more than just a few minutes. Penetration and thrusting meet deep needs in both genders.

But sometimes a man recognizes that his own orgasm is also more intense if he can delay it somewhat.

How can he—and she—delay his orgasm?

COCK RING

A metal, latex, or leather cock ring placed around the base of his penis can heighten sensation, delay orgasm, and, in some men, create a larger erection. It works by restricting the flow of blood out of his engorged penis. However, cock rings can bruise his flesh. They can also be dangerous if left on for longer than twenty minutes.

THE SQUEEZE TECHNIQUE

Masters and Johnson modeled their famous Squeeze Technique on the more elegant Taoist exercises described below. But the Squeeze is effective.

When he feels ejaculation is imminent but not inevitable, he withdraws. Either he or she lightly squeezes the head of his penis for several seconds. Then they can resume intercourse. The Squeeze can be repeated two or three times, if necessary.

ALTERNATING STIMULI

This is the simplest delaying method.

If you are highly aroused but not on the verge of ejaculation, stop thrusting and make love to your partner manually or orally. By alternating intercourse with other forms of lovemaking, most men can make lovemaking last longer. Sex therapists sometimes refer to this as the "stop-start" technique.

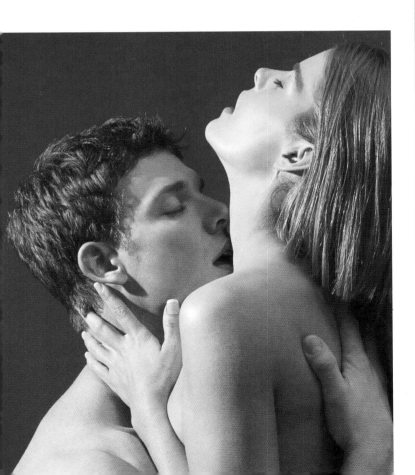

" Real talk "

"I ordered a cock ring online after seeing one used in a porn film," says Tony. "I thought it might be mildly exciting to wear it for a short time. My wife and I had played with nipple clamps. I thought it was the same kind of thing, an S/M toy. When I got the ring in the mail and read the accompanying material, I learned that it could actually help delay orgasm and sustain erection. I bought the damn little thing for a cheap thrill—and discovered that, used judiciously, it could help me prolong intercourse. Who says men don't read instructions?"

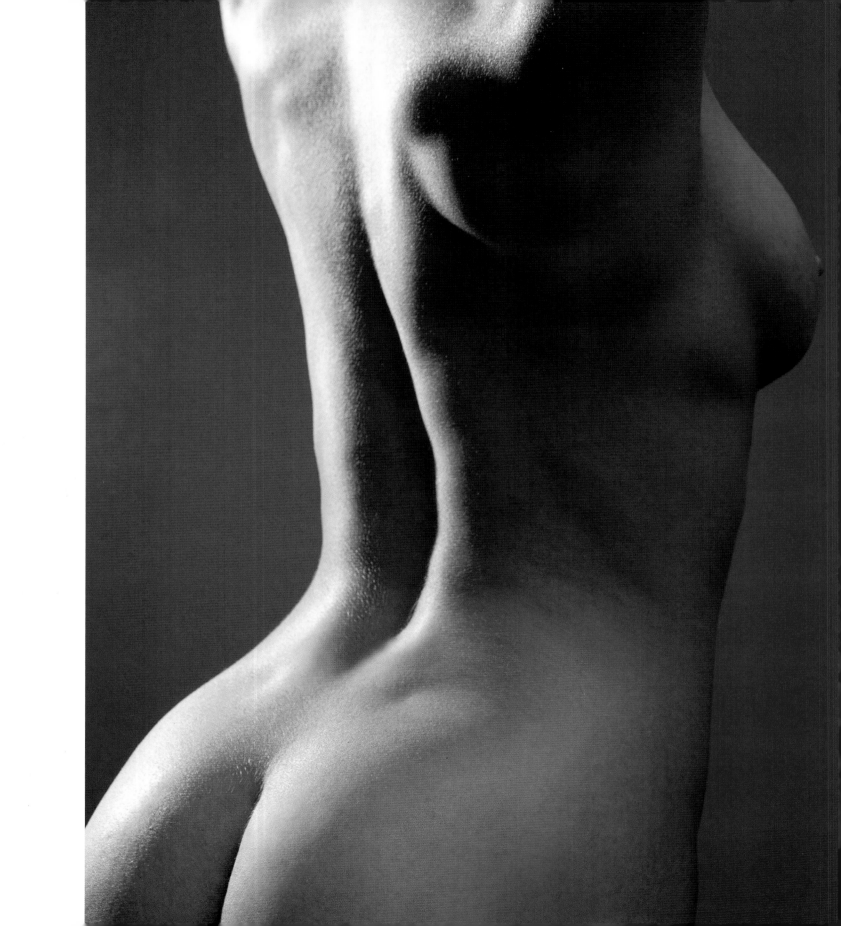

THE THREE-FINGER DRAW

Practiced in China for five thousand years, this technique is simple and, according to Mantak Chia, the leading teacher of Taoist sex techniques, "considerably effective." At the point of ejaculatory inevitability, use three curved fingers—his hand or hers—to apply pressure to the middle of the perineum. Experiment with pressure to see what works for him.

Generally speaking, that will be more pressure than she is likely to exert the first time she tries this.

THE BIG DRAW

This technique requires him to have a strong PC muscle.

"When you perfect the Big Draw," Mantak Chia says, "you won't need the Three-Finger Draw anymore."

He stops thrusting when he feels ejaculation is imminent and pulls back to approximately one inch of vaginal penetration. Do not withdraw entirely. Now he flexes his PC muscle and holds to a count of nine. (Or, as an alternative, flex the PC muscle nine times in rapid succession instead of holding the count.) Resume thrusting with shallow strokes.

"Real talk"

"I didn't think I needed an orgasm technique, because I usually had orgasms," says Jennie, "but I was game to try. The first few times I couldn't get it all working together, the breathing, the focusing, and the PC muscle. But then it did come together—and wow! I had a much stronger orgasm than normal. Now I use it all the time."

Marina says, "Everything had to be 'right' for me to have an orgasm—and as my husband kept pointing out, everything was seldom right. I needed to be relaxed and not stressed and have plenty of foreplay. Often I felt as if the sex started without me. I was present in body only.

"I was surprised at how quickly and easily the Orgasm Loop worked for me when I started masturbating with it. Using the Loop, I can have an orgasm anytime—without his spending an hour getting me there. He was shocked and delighted the first time I used it with him."

THE ORGASM LOOP

I developed the Orgasm Loop to give any woman a reliable means of having an orgasm anytime she wants one. Put simply, the Orgasm Loop is a revolutionary technique for reaching orgasm *anytime*, *every time*, and *multiple times*. It fuses cognitive feedback research on female orgasm and creative visualization therapy technique with Tantric breathing, PC flexing, *and*— a breakthrough concept—an adaptation of the same energy focus method that allows martial arts black belts to break boards, bricks, and blocks. Yet the Orgasm Loop is a simple technique that any woman can master quickly.

In years of interviewing women, I discovered that women have trouble reaching orgasm for three primary reasons:

1. **THEY DON'T KNOW WHAT THEY NEED** to reach orgasm—and perhaps have not yet had an orgasm.

   Masturbation therapy is the answer for these women. And the Loop makes that easy, even for women who are shy and inhibited.

2. **THEY DON'T KNOW HOW** to communicate their needs to their lovers.

   Get him involved in her Loop experience. He will be fascinated because it's new. And he won't feel that he's being criticized.

3. **THEY LOSE EROTIC FOCUS** during lovemaking because they are distracted by guilt/concern about children, chores, work—or body issues.

The Orgasm Loop was designed with these women in mind. They keep shutting down the erotic part of their brains and going back to the unfinished "to do" list. Or they obsess on their thighs or tummy or breasts they fear are beginning to sag. The Loop teaches them how to clear their minds and surrender to desire and arousal.

Why is "focus" primarily a woman's problem?

In women, the erotic mind–body connection is not as obvious as it is in men. Women don't see their arousal. So they need to learn how to visualize it.

Men are sexually simple; women are not. He gets an erection and he knows he wants to have sex if he can. The male erection–brain connection is strong. A woman's genitals don't always get the message to her brain—in part because the signs of female arousal are more subtle. Often she has sex without fully tapping into her arousal, making orgasm problematic. Or she allows herself to become distracted by body issues, performance concerns, stress, tension, worry—and loses her arousal, at least for a time, again making orgasm problematic.

Recent research has strengthened the conclusion most sexologists reached a long time ago: Sex for women begins in the brain. If she doesn't get her head into sex, it never really happens to her—no matter what her lover does.

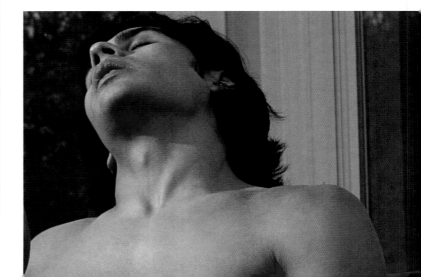

Why does the Orgasm Loop work?

It teaches a woman how to visualize her arousal and then focus all her sexual energy on achieving orgasm in a three-stage process.

The more she visualizes arousal, the more aroused she becomes—until orgasm is easy, as inevitable as it is for a man.

How does it work?

The three stages are mental arousal, energy focus; and physical moves, including breathing, PC flexing, and clitoral stimulation via hand, mouth, vibrator, or penis.

Technique Tip

THE ORGASM LOOP

Mental Arousal
Close your eyes, clear your mind of distractions, and visualize your arousal.

Some women may visualize their genitalia—lips swelling, moisture forming, the color changing to deeper pink. Other women may visualize a flower, perhaps an orchid. (The sensual flower paintings of Georgia O'Keefe can be an inspiration.) Some women may see arousal as a color, perhaps pink or red—or saffron yellow, the color of the goddess in Hindu mythology. A beach at sunset can be an arousal image.

Find the image that represents arousal to you and focus on it every time you use the Orgasm Loop. This image must become your mental erotic mantra. Focus to the extent that no other image enters your mind.

Note: Eye contact with your lover during the cognitive conditioning phase will slow the process. Keep eyes closed during kissing/foreplay.

Energy Focus
When you are conscious of nothing but arousal, turn your focus inward.

Focus on a spot just below your navel (the inner chi, if we want to get technical). Breathe deeply and slowly and imagine that little spot of energy glowing and growing. Move it down into your genitals with your breath.

Hold that energy in place.

Now imagine a fiery coil of sexual energy located at the base of your spine (kundalini or life force). Uncoil it and move it into your genitals. Feel the undulating coiling energy circling around and through the spot of glowing energy.

You have moved your body's energy into your genitals, particularly the clitoris. And you are experiencing heightened sensitivity to touch now because you have created a physiological response in your body. Your heartbeat is accelerated. Your body temperature is rising. You feel more alive, more sensuous with the heat. And the blood flow concentrated in your genitals is making them incredibly sensitive.

Physical Moves

1. While maintaining your energy focus, use breathing to intensify the mind–genital connection. Imagine you are breathing fire in a circle, inhaling it up from your genitals throughout your body and exhaling from your mouth. . . . Keep doing this in circular fashion. (See "Fire Breathing," page 36.)

2. Once you have created a circle of fire, flex your PC muscle in time with your breathing. Tighten it as you breathe in; loosen as you breathe out. The combination of controlled breathing and energy focusing creates heat. You literally move that heat in and out of your body in an exciting circle as you Fire Breathe. Like any form of deep breathing, it increases the oxygen level in the blood. And it forces more blood into your genital area.

   Keep up the Fire Breathing during intercourse. Don't worry if you lose a cycle or two. Just pick it up again, especially at the point of orgasm, because it intensifies orgasm.

3. Apply clitoral stimulation—either orally or manually or by positioning yourself in intercourse to make the hot spot connection between the shaft of the penis and the clitoris. Very little stimulation will be necessary at this point to achieve orgasm.

And you can have more orgasms simply by maintaining the focus and the breathing instead of relaxing after the orgasm.

Try the Orgasm Loop alone during masturbation at least once or twice before incorporating it into lovemaking.

The Bigger Orgasms: Multiple, Extended, and Whole-Body Orgasms

Everything else is supersized these days. Why not orgasms?

No matter what the catchy title says on some books, you can't make them last an hour—unless you start counting at the first foreplay tingle. But you can make them longer, stronger, more frequent and intense.

MULTIPLE ORGASMS

All women are capable of having multiple orgasms, though probably fewer than a third of women do have them—and even fewer have them on a regular basis. Unlike men, women don't need a refractory period to "recover" from one orgasm before they can have another. If a woman wants to have multiple orgasms, she can learn how to do it.

There are four types of multiple orgasms experienced by women. Each can be achieved via intercourse, oral or manual stimulation (including the G-spot), or a combination thereof. They are:

Compounded single orgasms

Each orgasm is distinct, separated by sufficient time so that prior arousal and tension have substantially resolved between orgasms.

Sequential multiples

Orgasms are fairly close together—anywhere from one to ten minutes apart—with little interruption in sexual stimulation or level of arousal.

Serial multiples

Orgasms are separated by seconds, or up to two minutes, with no—or barely any—interruption in stimulation or diminishment of arousal.

Blended multiples

A mix of two or more of the above types. Very often women who are multiply orgasmic experience more than one type of multiple orgasm during a lovemaking session.

You can encourage multiple orgasms by using the Orgasm Loop or the following techniques:

> ## "Real talk"
>
> Jeremy says, "You really have to get your lover involved in this technique. She has to hold still while you remain one inch inside her. That's not going to work if she wants to have an orgasm. If you do work out the timing with her—and you've done those damned Kegels until you have the muscle power for it—the Big Draw is awesome. I can do it twice during intercourse. I have an orgasm that feels like it's blowing the top of my head off at the same time it's curling my toes. This isn't easy, but it is worth the time you put into Kegels and practicing the Big Draw."

Technique Tip

ALTERNATING STIMULI

During lovemaking, alternate stimuli—manual, oral, thrusting—to achieve multiple orgasms. The first one or two orgasms, for example, may be via oral or manual stimulation. Women who do have multiples are more likely to have them if the lovemaking doesn't begin with intercourse.

Why?

Generally, it takes women longer to reach orgasm via intercourse—unless they've already had an orgasm.

Here's the ideal scenario: He gives you the first orgasm via cunnilingus. Oral sex more fully (and quickly) arouses the female genitalia than any other form of stimuli. Then he adds manual stroking of your clitoral area, labia, and P spot as you're having the orgasm. After you experience a second or third one, he inserts his penis while maintaining manual stimulation with one hand.

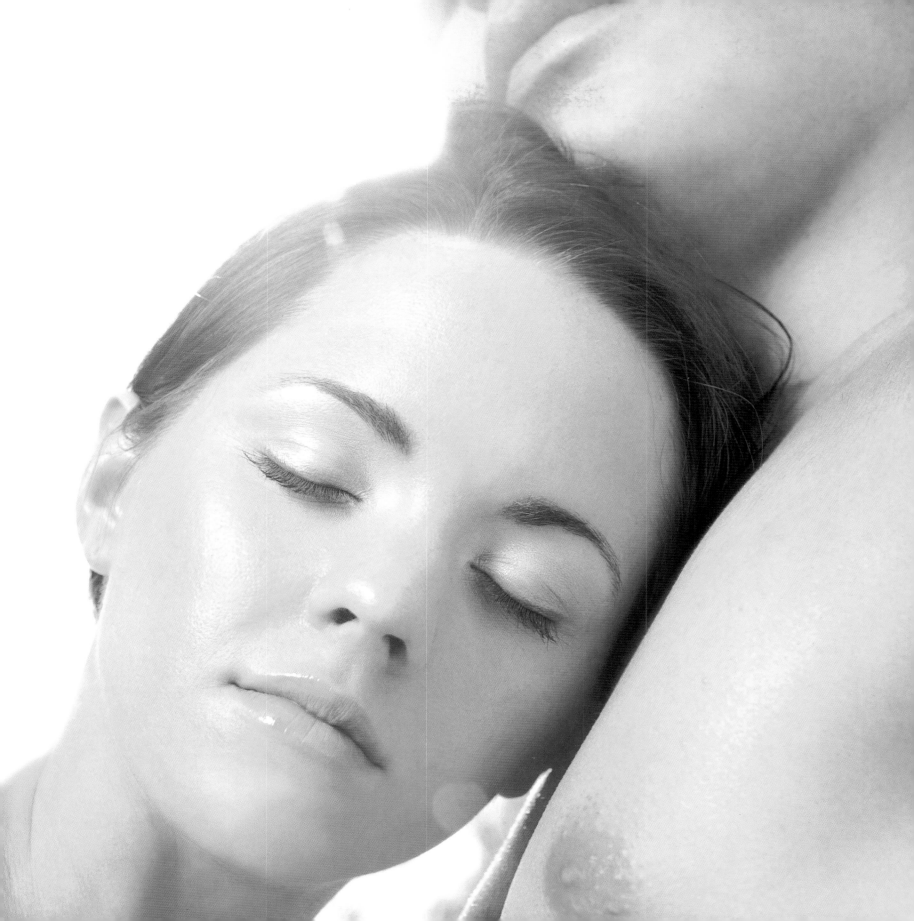

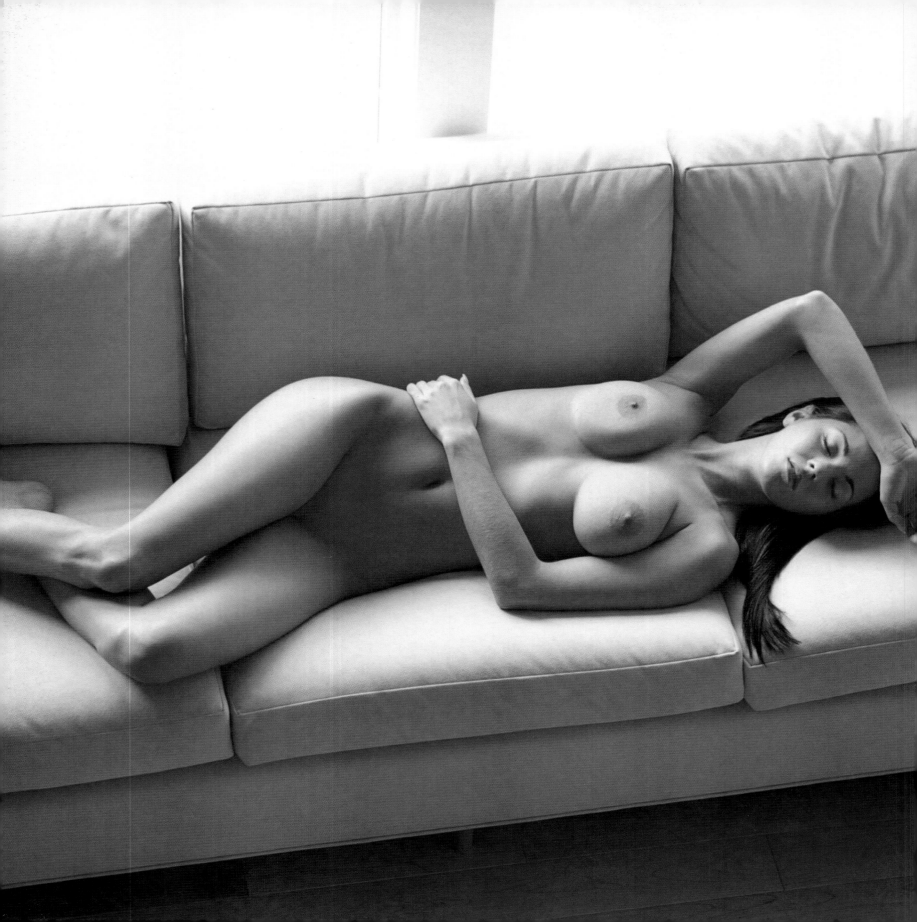

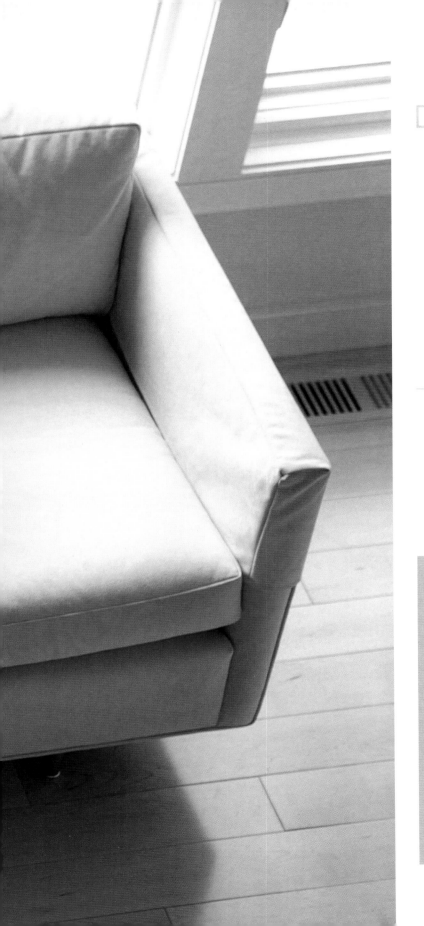

HANDS-ON INTERCOURSE

Women who aren't comfortable touching themselves during intercourse are less likely to experience multiple orgasms. Most women do need that additional touch to reach orgasm. Or they need a lot of time. Multiples occur when the first orgasm happens quickly and easily.

Stroke yourself during cunnilingus or intercourse—or take his hand and show him how you want to be stroked. (Think about it: You are combining the high manual stimulation you get in masturbation with everything your lover can do for you. Yes!) When you feel the orgasm coming, don't stop the stimulation as you probably do now.

Continue stroking. Feel another orgasm building up behind the first one.

" Real talk "

"That first oral orgasm opens the door to more orgasms for me in a way that a first orgasm via other means just doesn't," says Lisa. "Maybe it's all in my head, but I feel wider concentric waves of pleasure throughout my clitoris and vagina from an oral orgasm. If he keeps going—with his tongue or hand or a combination of both—I keep coming. Then when he enters me, it feels like his penis is stirring those sensations up and shooting them out into my body. I can come several times if he really pays attention to what he's doing."

G-SPOT MULTIPLES

Some women can have multiple orgasms only when they are receiving both clitoral and vaginal stimulation in the area of the-G spot. Here's how he can do that for her:

He uses his fingers to stimulate the front wall of her vagina while he's performing cunnilingus, or:

He (or she) stimulates her clitoris during intercourse in a position that gives her G-spot stimulation.

Technique Tip

THE FLICKERING FLAME

Some women will have multiple orgasms only through prolonged and expert cunnilingus. Here's one way of doing it for her:

Pretend the tip of your tongue is a candle flame. In your mind's eye, see that flame flickering in the wind. Move your tongue rapidly around the sides of her clitoris, above and below it, across the tiny shaft, as the candle flame moves.

When she starts to orgasm, lick the sides of her clitoris in slow, even strokes. As you feel the orgasm subside, go back to the flame until she begins to come again.

Finally, some women cannot say that one method or another will create multiple orgasms for them. Other factors have more influence. It may be her mood or her hormonal balance or the quality of her fantasies before sex—or how she is feeling about her partner. You can't discount the importance of emotions. Some women who are capable of multiple orgasms may have them only with a special man.

During lovemaking, can they tell that this will be the night for multiples?

Yes, they probably can—once the first orgasm begins.

"Real talk"

"I can't have multiple orgasms unless I am stroking my clitoris—or he is—during intercourse or cunnilingus," says Stacey. "I can come again and again if I am getting a specific kind of touch, the way I touch myself when I masturbate. I use my finger or thumb to make circles around my clitoris. If that is combined with shallow thrusting in intercourse, it drives me wild. The orgasms start. I keep having them even after he is thrusting hard."

A COUPLE'S STORY

"I know I'm going to have multiples when the first orgasm doesn't feel like a complete release," she says. "I've become aroused to the point where it will take several orgasms to release the tension. My lover can't see when it is going to, or could possibly, happen. I look the same on the outside—sweaty, flushed, dilated pupils, all the signs of arousal. It's not as if I have a pop-up thermometer inside that jumps out and says, 'She's hotter than usual today.'"

He says, "If she would signal to me that she is in a state where she could have multiple orgasms, I would pay attention to that. I would keep stimulating her through orgasm and help her get to the next and the next.

"She leaves me out of her orgasms, except at the end, when she pulls me to her in a sort of grateful embrace. I don't know why men think they give women orgasms. We don't. Women take their orgasms or they withhold them from us. They aren't waiting for the gift-wrapped orgasm to be handed over. "

"I am not always open to the intensity of having multiple orgasms," she says. "It leaves me feeling vulnerable, somehow. I don't always like the feeling. But I want to get over that. I think I can with this man. He's more in tune with me than anyone I have known. We are more honest with each other."

"We have conversations like I haven't had with another woman," he says. "And multiple orgasms are a conversation, even if she's the one talking and I'm the one trying to listen and figure it all out. The little gasp and moan she makes at the end of everyday orgasms get caught in her throat when she's having multiples. That's my first clue.

"Feeling and watching her have multiples is an awesome experience. I really am in awe of her. I almost don't blame her for being a little secretive, holding her information close, and letting me know that I have to figure out the way in here. She's like a high priestess of sex—and I am the guy at her feet who wants to learn and be given more access."

"That will happen," she says.

What about men?

Well, that depends on both the man and how he defines orgasm. Typically, male orgasm is equated with ejaculation. Men cannot have multiple ejaculations within a span of a few minutes, but some men can have multiple orgasms—as they define multiple orgasms—in that time period.

How?

They experience the contractions without ejaculating.

This is an esoteric technique, disparaged by some mainstream therapists and sexologists and not likely to be workable for very young men or for the man who has only occasional sex. Basically, it's a repackaging of four-thousand-year-old Taoist techniques for ejaculatory control. (See page 198 for more.) Don't be discouraged if you can't make this happen, but here are the basics, if you want to try:

Technique Tip

HIS MALE MULTIPLES— THE "NO EJACULATION" ORGASM

Learn to control the sphincter muscle.

Strengthen the PC muscle by practicing Kegel exercises. (See page 36.)

When you feel you are about to ejaculate, attempt to hold it back by squeezing the sphincter and PC muscles. This will be difficult, even a little painful, but if you persevere, you may be able to delay ejaculation for several minutes. Practice while masturbating.

Without quite realizing how you did it, one day you may experience the contractions and pleasurable sensations of orgasm—without ejaculating.

Continued stimulation via intercourse, oral, or manual means will produce multiple orgasms without ejaculation.

FEMALE EJACULATION

Like male multiples, female ejaculation is something you either believe in or don't. There's not a lot of science backing any claims.

Female ejaculation isn't exactly a technique. Some devotees of goddess cults claim that every woman can learn to ejaculate during orgasm. But that's a minority opinion. The more common response is: women—*ejaculate?*

Western sex experts generally dismiss female ejaculation as either a myth or a gush of fluid composed of urine and copious vaginal secretions. There is no doubt that it isn't the female equivalent of seminal fluid. Some women do ejaculate—or squirt, if you prefer—fluid upon orgasm, especially a G-spot orgasm.

According to one very small school of thought, the fluid might be produced by the Skene's glands, a collection of several masses of tissue strung out along the urinary tract. These glands don't even exist in all women. Medical researcher Josephine Lowndes Sevely says that in women who do have Skene's glands, the fluid produced is neither urine nor vaginal secretions.

Few women claim to have ejaculated. Many of those who do are embarrassed by the squirting fluids. Hint to men: Don't ask her if she's peeing on you.

"Real talk"

"Men think I am peeing on them," says Cassidy. "Ejaculation happens for me only when I am really aroused—by a man who has stimulated my AFE Zone and my G-spot. To me that indicates it's an excess of vaginal fluid that explodes out of my vagina in a rush when I reach orgasm. I love the intensity of the big wet orgasms, but I wish they didn't leave the man and the bed so wet."

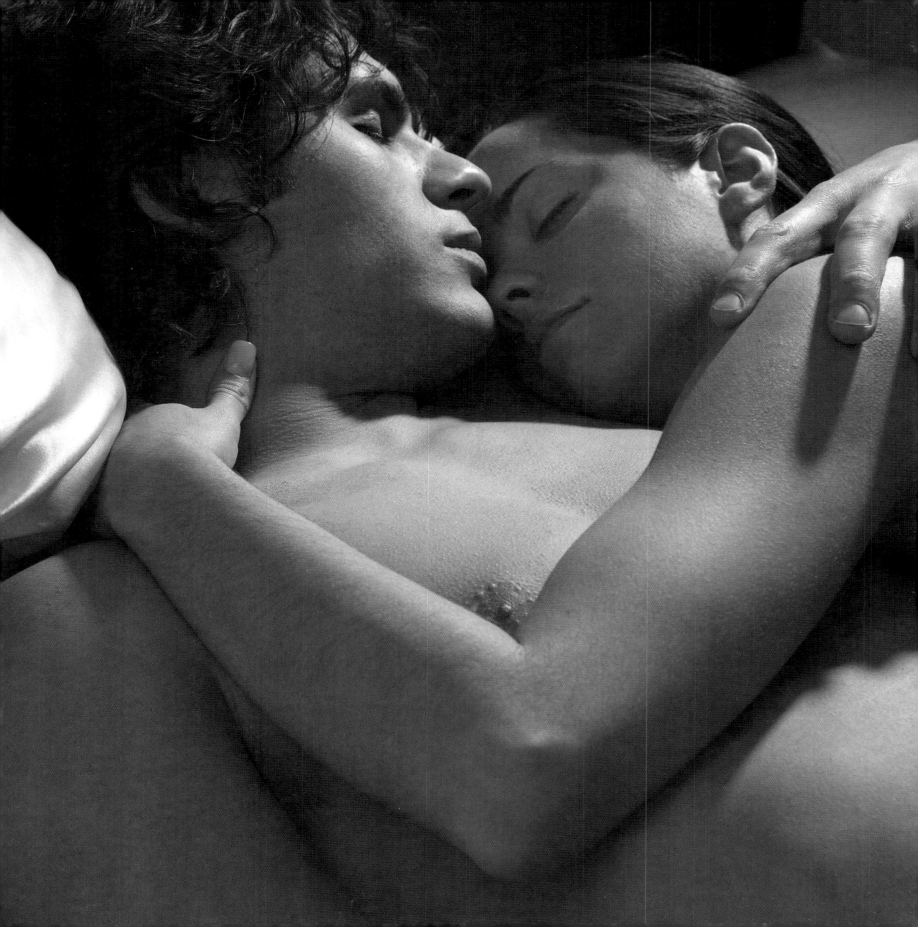

A COUPLE'S STORY

Jane and Mark met at a weekend Tantric sex workshop at Canyon Ranch. She was married to Anthony and he was married to Cynthia at the time. Both couples were "working on the relationship" with their spouses prior to recognizing the relationship was over and filing for divorce.

Mark caught Jane's eye at the breakfast discussion group. The Tantric guru asked couples to share their "night-before sex stories." Mark didn't believe the tales reported by a few couples, dutifully weaving in the techniques taught in the previous day's workshop on orgasm. He was laughing inside when he glanced at Jane.

He knew she was laughing, too.

They went for a walk alone the following day. It was just a walk, nothing more. They didn't even hold hands. Jane said her marriage wasn't going to be saved by Tantra. Mark said his wasn't, either, that he knew his wife had a lover.

"She brought me to sex camp," he said, laughing derisively, "hoping I would turn into her lover overnight. I didn't. She's probably on the phone with him right now."

"I brought Anthony to sex camp, too," Jane said ruefully. "Really, I brought us both here. Looking for a miracle. How silly is that?"

They exchanged phone numbers and promised to call if he got to Boston or she to New York City.

A year and two divorces later, he found her phone number in his flight bag and called her.

"Where are you?" she asked.

"At LaGuardia airport," he lied. "Do you have time for dinner tonight?"

She said, "Yes." He threw some things into an overnight bag, dashed to the airport, and grabbed a shuttle flight to New York. When he walked into her favorite Indian restaurant, his bag over his shoulder, she was sitting at the bar. She saw him and laughed out loud. He went to her and kissed her neck.

They talked and laughed and touched and generally enjoyed each other so much that he didn't think to worry about whether or not he remembered any miracle technique from that Tantric weekend, until she excused herself and went to the ladies' room. He watched her walk away from him, his eyes on her slender waist and the full rise of her buttocks. His penis, hard for some time, pushed against the fabric of his trousers. She stopped, turned around, and smiled at him. Something in her smile told him she knew what he had inside his pants.

An hour later, his bag was on her bedroom floor and he was in her bed. In a tangle of wet mouths and hands, legs and arms, he knew something important. He hadn't failed this woman as a lover—and he wasn't going to fail her, either. With his fingers, he stroked her swollen, wet labia and made his way to her clitoris. He couldn't remember where he had learned what to do.

He remembered only to do it. Right. This time. He felt the pulse of her body surging through her clitoris. She throbbed between his fingers. He couldn't wait to take his mouth there.

EXTENDED ORGASMS

If you study Tantric sex, you will come across the concept of "sexual ecstasy" or "high sex." That simply means extending the time that orgasm lasts and expanding orgasm beyond the genitals. Doing these things, of course, is not all that simple and takes a little practice. Learn how to extend your orgasms during masturbation.

And the really good news: Men can enjoy extended orgasms, too.

Technique Tip

HER EXTENDED ORGASM

Masturbate in a comfortable position using the Orgasm Loop on (page 149). Keep the arousal image and the Fire Breathing going continuously rather than stopping when orgasm begins, so that your orgasm extends (and likely becomes multiples).

You can both use these techniques during lovemaking. Extended orgasms are more likely to occur when you have time for slow, languorous lovemaking—the kind of sex that keeps you feeling "on the verge" for a long time. This is a "slowie," not a quickie.

A good "staying on the edge" position is the X (see page 125), or scissors (see page 248), because he can sustain that position with a semierection. Breathe deeply, move slowly, and use your hands to stroke each other, working upward from your genitals.

Resist the temptation to thrust hard and fast when you reach that agonizing point of being "almost there." The longer you stay on the verge, the longer the orgasm will be.

HIS EXTENDED ORGASM

Masturbate without ejaculating for as long as you can. Use the stop-and-start method, or change strokes when you feel ejaculation is imminent.

Count the contractions you experience during ejaculation, normally between three and eight. Note the level and order of intensity. Typically, the strongest contraction will be the first one.

The next time you masturbate, again delay ejaculation as long as possible.

When you do ejaculate, flex your PC muscle. Then continue stimulating your penis very slowly while squeezing throughout the ejaculation—effectively pushing the sensations of orgasm on longer.

WHOLE-BODY ORGASMS

Occasionally an orgasm is both intense and diffuse. The tremors seem to radiate from the genitals to the far reaches of the body's extremities. You feel it blowing out the top of your head and out through your toes.

Some people experience whole-body orgasms only when they have a strong emotional connection to their partners, others when they are feeling particularly sensual or sexual or both. The whole-body orgasm is most likely the result of intense connection on three levels—emotional, sensual, and sexual—though, again, nothing is true for everyone. Consider the levels to be separate doors, three possible ways into the whole-body orgasm.

Imagine orgasmic waves getting bigger and bigger as they wash over your body. You can make it happen.

HER WHOLE-BODY ORGASM

Masturbate in a comfortable position.

As soon as you become highly aroused, use your other hand to massage your vulva, inner thighs, and groin with light, shallow strokes. Imagine that you are spreading arousal throughout those areas. Continue the massage during your orgasm, imagining you are spreading the orgasms into your body.

Next time you masturbate, apply the Orgasm Loop technique and the manual spreading. Now apply this combined-technique method in lovemaking.

HIS WHOLE-BODY ORGASM

You need a strong PC muscle for this.

During masturbation (and later intercourse), stop thrusting when you feel ejaculation is imminent. Flex the PC muscle and hold to a count of nine. Or try flexing nine times in rapid succession instead of holding the count. Now resume thrusting.

EXTRAGENITAL ORGASMS

One to three percent of women—and almost no men—can reach orgasm without genital stimulation. When it does occur, extragenital orgasm usually follows an orgasm (or more) triggered the old-fashioned way, by the genitals. A highly orgasmic woman, for example, can reach the third, fourth, or fifth orgasm having her breasts or nipples stroked, sucked, pinched, pulled, or massaged. Some women at that point can even come by squeezing their thighs together.

This is not so much a talent—or a learned response—as a blessing.

But this technique can encourage extragenital orgasm in women who are orgasmic in most of their lovemaking encounters—and have also experienced multiple orgasms. The directions are for him.

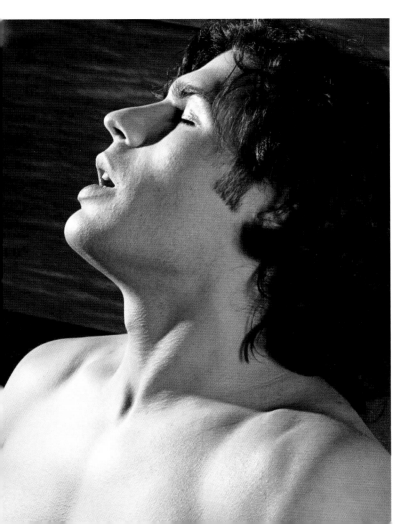

┌─────────────────────────────────────┐
│   **Technique Tip**   │
└─────────────────────────────────────┘

TAKING HER OVER THE TOP

Caress your lover's genitals orally and manually until she is near orgasm.

Now shift your hands and mouth to congenital areas; for example, kiss her mouth, throat, breasts, inner thighs.

Go back to genital caresses.

When she is near orgasm again, move your hands and mouth to other parts of her body.

Alternate from genital to nongenital stimulation until she is so aroused—in a state of hypersensitivity—that you can bring her to orgasm; for example, by stroking and licking her inner thighs or sucking one nipple while massaging the other breast. The orgasm will feel as if it starts in the clitoris—but expands to a whole-body orgasm, with particular tingling in the nongenital site of the triggering caress.

" Real talk "

Wesley says, "My first whole-body orgasm took me by surprise. My wife and I had been practicing the techniques, but I had little expectation they would work for me. We'd spent a long weekend in bed. I was drained, yet also oddly energized. That orgasm blew out the top of my head and the soles of my feet.

"It was almost an out-of-body experience.

"I told her, 'Honey, the earth moved.'"

THE PERINEUM (OR THE MALE G-SPOT) ORGASM

Whenever I give testers a perineum technique,
I get back the widest range of responses imaginable.
A little perineum massage makes some men crazy, has
little effect on others, and leaves many confused and
a few even repulsed and ready to defend their refusal
to have a male G-spot orgasm with weapons at thirty
paces. So. This is the technique. It works for many,
but not all. Try it—and if you don't like it, that's okay.

" Real talk "

"Sometimes I feel the tremors all over my body during orgasm," says Debra. "First, my body goes taut. It's like my breasts and nipples and vaginal walls are expanding. They feel bigger and bigger. My whole body is alive and aroused and quivering. The orgasms start in my genitals, like waves in my clitoris, spreading out to my labia, into my vagina, deep inside the walls. They reverberate there and grow bigger and spill outside until I feel them throughout my body, even in the tips of my fingers and toes.

"I see colors flashing, bright primary colors. It's a transcendent experience that lifts me outside my body and puts me back down again."

Technique Tip

HIS PERINEUM ORGASM

Excite your lover to the point of orgasm via oral and manual stimulation to his genitals. (Don't neglect testicles.) Stop the stimulation. Repeat.

When you notice him writhing almost in pain, hold his thighs apart and lower your mouth to his perineum. Flick your tongue rapidly back and forth on that area. Now insert a finger or a thumb and press into his perineum—gauging the pressure by his response—as you continue flicking your tongue.

If he has an orgasm this way, it will send powerful vibrations through his body.

If he can't have an orgasm this way, he will either thrust his penis into your mouth or pull you up on top of him. And there's nothing wrong with his having an orgasm either way.

Technique Tip

SPONTANEOUS ORGASM

Dr. Annie Sprinkle, famed sexologist and performance artist, teaches a no-hands, or "spontaneous," orgasm.

Begin Fire Breathing. Keep doing it until you are highly aroused, probably ten to fifteen minutes.

Add PC flexing. Flex the muscle in time with Fire Breathing.

And don't worry if you can't reach orgasm this way. You can get very aroused. Orgasm will follow by more conventional means.

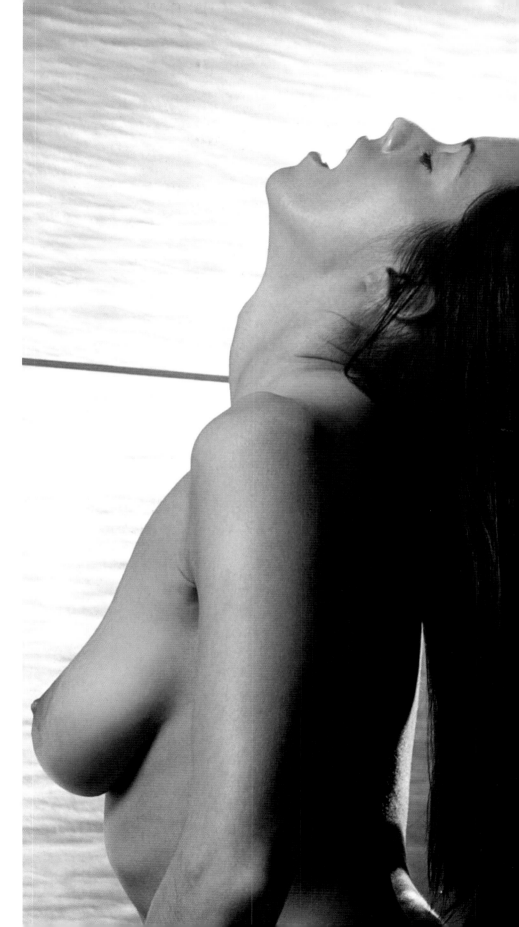

Special Orgasm Experiences

When you have time for making love all day, you can have the kind of sex that keeps you feeling on the edge for long periods of time. She will have one or more orgasms before the extended play begins. He will likely have an early orgasm, too.

You can turn extended lovemaking into extraordinary orgasm experiences, one for him and one for her. These techniques require a high degree of erotic control, amazing PC muscles, and a love of sex play.

"Some women can 'think themselves off'; that is, fantasize to orgasm. Women have a huge orgasmic potential that is sadly not always realized."

— Gina Ogden, Ph.D.
Author of *Women Who Love Sex: An Inquiry into the Expanding Spirit of Women's Erotic Experience*

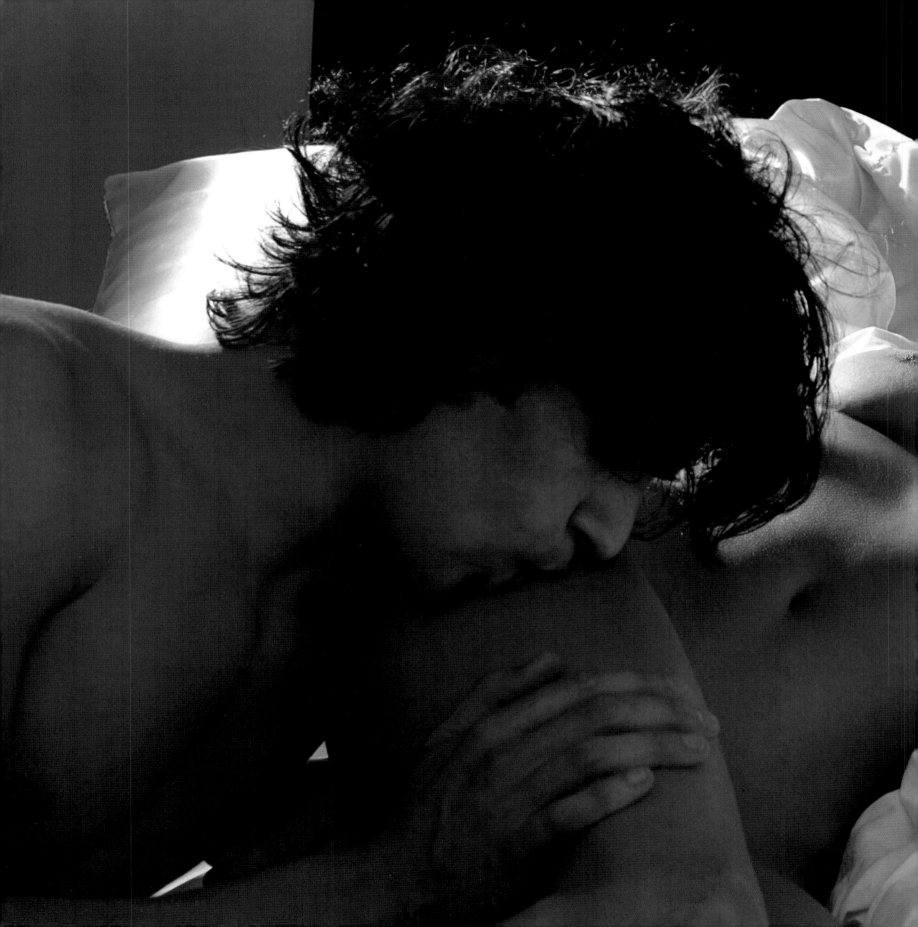

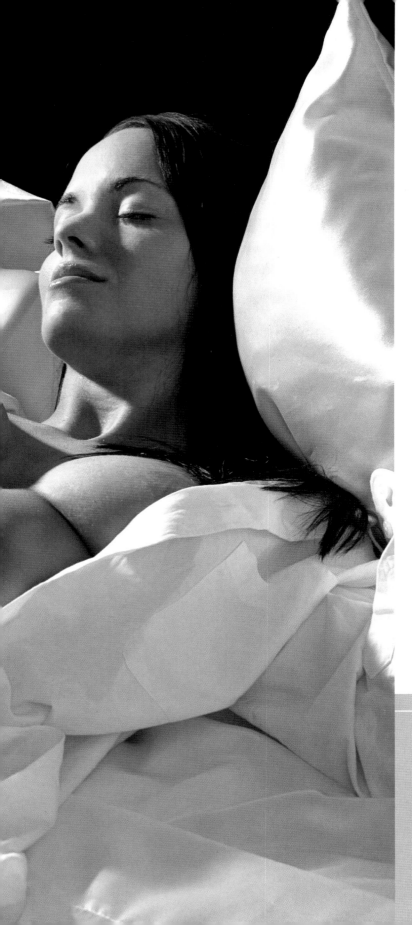

KAREZZA

An Italian word that means "caress," karezza is a technique adapted from ancient erotic teachings via a minister. The name was given to a supposedly new (at the time) technique developed in 1883 by an American physician, Alice Bunker Stockham. She actually borrowed it from a pamphlet on birth control written by a founding member of the Oneida Community, a minister who adapted it from a blend of Tantric and Taoist teachings.

Stockham had her patients prepare for karezza by reading uplifting writings, such as the poems of Elizabeth Barrett Browning and the philosophy of Ralph Waldo Emerson. And she thought lovers should hold the position for an hour. "Discuss the writings you have read during this period of tranquil sexual union," she lectured. (One may assume she was a virgin.)

Karezza prolongs intercourse and encourages extended orgasm. For the jaded sophisticate, it is a new way to make love.

Dramatically limit his genital movement in either the female superior or the side-by-side position. He does not move inside her unless he becomes flaccid, and then he executes only a few shallow thrusts to revive his erection. But he can—and should!—stroke her breasts and clitoris.

She is in charge of movement, including thrusting her hips against him or contracting her PC muscle around his penis.

No matter how excited he gets, he thrusts only enough to sustain his erection.

He holds their lovemaking embrace until she has achieved at least one and preferably more orgasms.

When a man lightly caresses a woman's body—with his hands or lips—it can be erotically stimulating, as well as a sensual way to infuse intimacy into the act of making love.

KABBAZAH

Thousands of years ago in the Middle East, at a time when that part of the world was not dominated by religious extremists, a woman who had mastered the art of "pompoir," control of the PC muscle during intercourse, was called a *kabazzah*, or "one who holds." Kabazzahs were the best prostitutes. Their lifestyle was equivalent to that enjoyed today by the most expensive call girls, such as the European and American women who service the sexual needs of rich Arabs at their lavish parties.

An extended orgasm just for him, Kabbazah (the technique) has long been a specialty of Asian, particularly in modern times the Japanese, prostitutes. In their way, they are carrying on the sacred sex tradition of the Indian temple prostitutes. (I am referring to professional courtesans, women who are well trained in the erotic arts and have chosen their career, not the underage girls sold into sexual slavery or forced into it by poverty.) American soldiers in World War II and Vietnam discovered Kabbazah on R & R leaves. This discovery was neither reported in the mainstream press nor immortalized in musicals such as *South Pacific*.

The requirements for Kabbazah are:

- He must be in a relaxed and receptive state of mind and body. His passivity is crucial.

- She must have a talented vagina. A woman can't perform Kabbazah unless she has achieved mastery of her PC muscle through Kegels for *at least* a period of three weeks to a month.

Some positions are better than others for Kabbazah. The female superior and sitting positions work best for most couples. But do experiment.

She stimulates her lover until he is just erect, not highly aroused. Then she inserts his penis.

He does not move his penis at all. Never. Not once.

She also strives for no pelvic movement, confining movement as much as possible to her PC muscle.

Kiss and caress each other freely.

Flex her PC muscle in varying patterns until she feels his penis throbbing—indicating an intense level of arousal—which should occur approximately ten to fifteen minutes into Kabbazah.

She times her contractions to the throbbing of his penis, clenching and releasing in time with him.

He will experience a longer, more intense orgasm than normal.

And after his orgasm, she can flex her PC muscle like crazy and have an orgasm of her own.

"Real talk"

Andre says, "I enjoy perineum stimulation. I like to be pressed harder than she likes to press. I've learned to put my finger over hers and show her how hard to go. The combination of tongue and finger on my perineum gave me a wonderful, strong orgasm."

A MAN'S STORY

Michael served in Afghanistan as a fighter pilot. On leave in Southeast Asia, he sought out a woman who could practice Kabbazah, something he'd read about in the journal of a Vietnam war hero published online. Back in those days, many women schooled in sexual arts might have had some knowledge of Kabbazah.

Times change. Now most women are proficient at fellatio and are willing to submit to kinky practices. But Kabbazah is an esoteric, nearly lost art.

On his last day of leave in Bangkok, Michael was introduced to Rae, a Eurasian woman in her mid-forties, not the lithe girl of his fantasies. But she was, according to the concierge who put them together, "the one to know Kabbazah." He decided to go home with her.

In her elegant apartment rich with fabric and art from India, Morocco, and Africa, he relaxed in the bath she drew for him, sipped her vintage champagne, and began to relax. Whatever, he thought. If he just got a nice massage, he would be okay with the experience.

Her naked body was trim and toned, her pubis waxed, every inch of her oiled and perfumed. He forgot she was nearly two decades his senior as he settled into her sumptuous bed and waited for whatever came next. She took his penis into her hands and it sprang to life.

"Lie still and do not move," she said softly. "You must leave everything to me."

Rae climbed on top of Michael and repeated her admonishment: "Remember, do not move. I play man's role in the movement."

He complied. Not moving would have been harder if he hadn't spent the previous four nights masturbating himself to sleep in his hotel room. He was able to lie still, his eyes closed, his focus entirely on the experience. She moved very little. He vaguely wondered if he would fall asleep, if that were all there was to this "esoteric art."

Then he felt the flexing begin around his penis. She clenched him in her muscle—and released. Clenched and released. Slowly. Surely. He swelled up inside her to what felt like the size of a monster appendage.

The sensations were like nothing he'd ever felt. He'd never been inside a woman the way he was inside Rae. Toward the end, she was not moving her body at all. Only her muscle moved, grasping his penis in an erotic grip so powerful and arousing that he almost believed he had died and gone to heaven.

She engaged him with her muscle—induced in him a long, slow orgasm that lasted so long. Afterward she let him sleep. He had tears in his eyes when he left her.

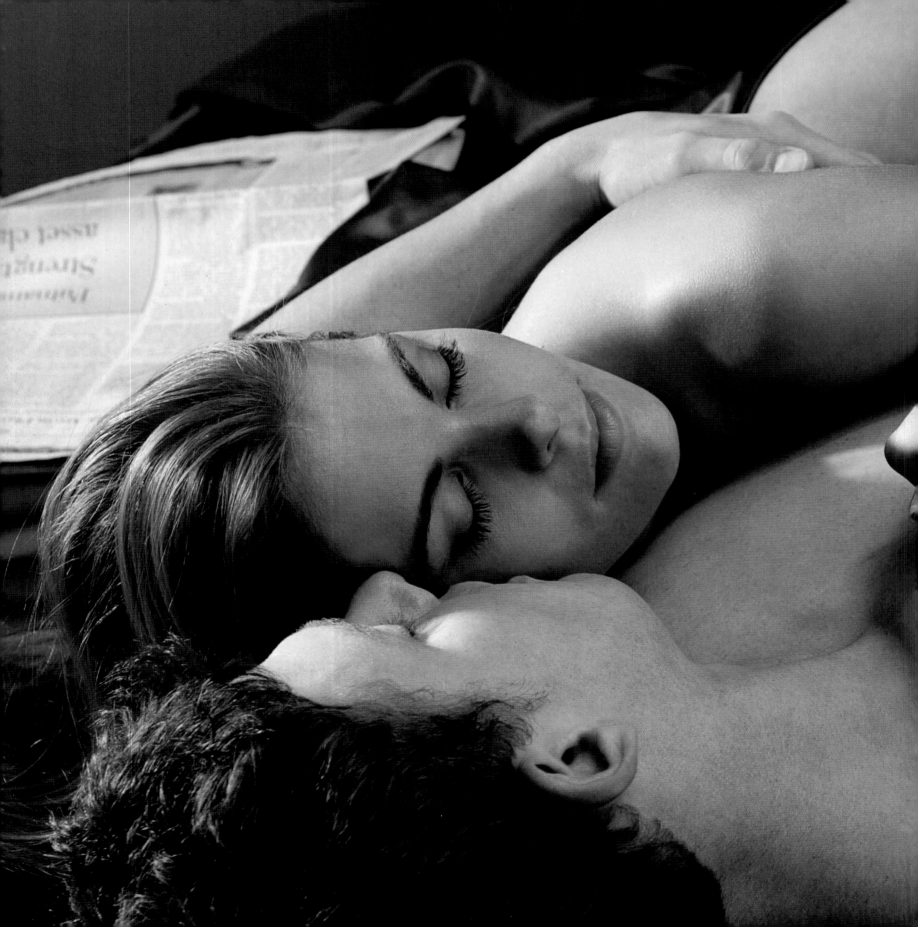

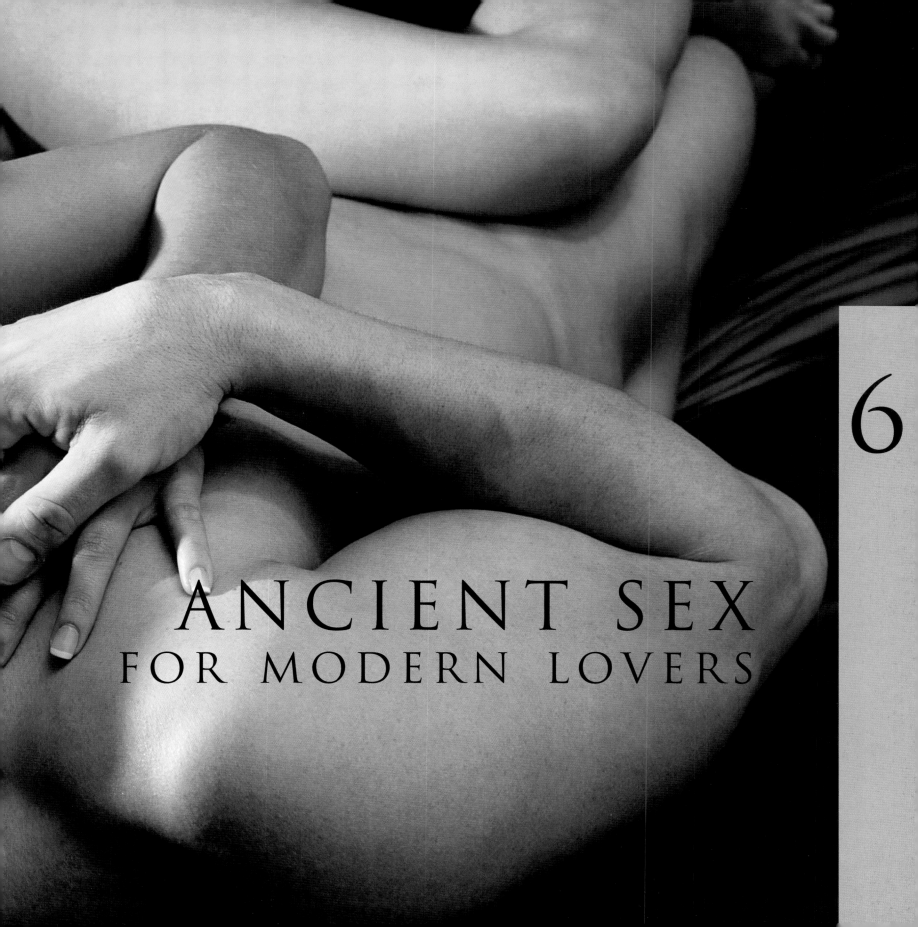

ANCIENT SEX
FOR MODERN LOVERS

6

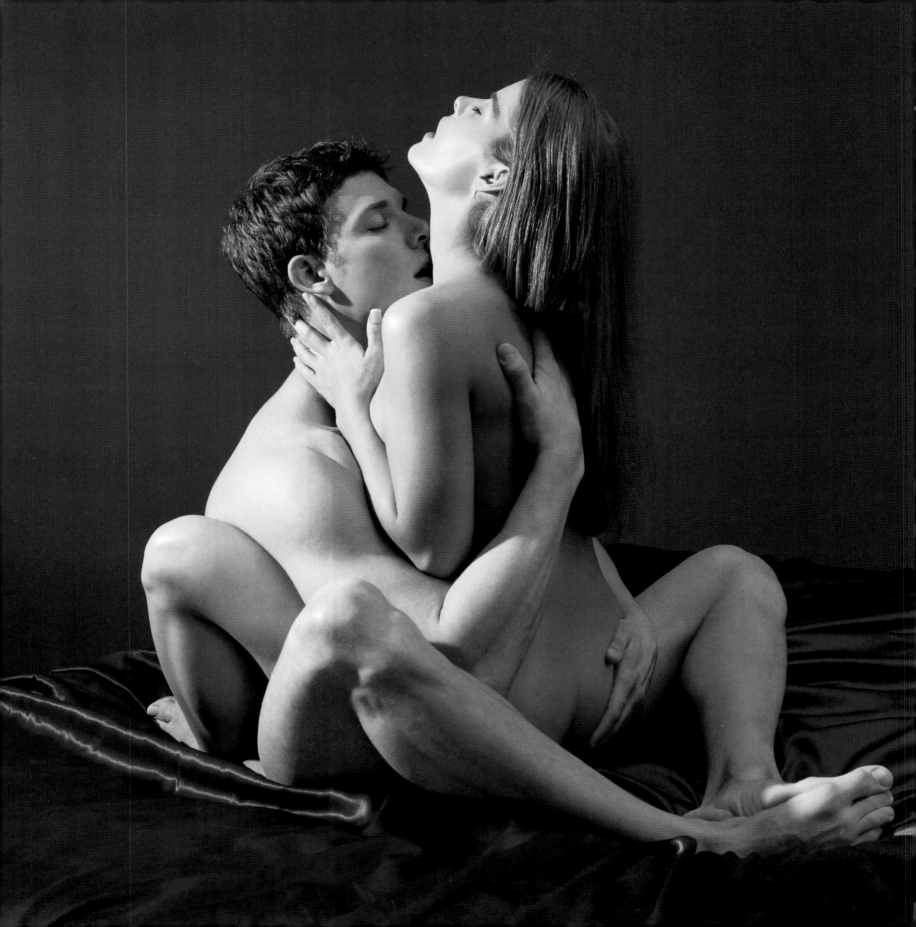

SACRED SEXUALITY

———

"Tantra, even Tantra Lite, gives both men and women some techniques—

eye contact, sensual massage, breathing rituals—

to help them slow down and get beyond goal-oriented sex.

Men get beyond their penises and the urge to take over the woman's

pleasure; women often take more initiative."

— Margot Anand
Author, *The Art of Sexual Ecstasy*

As you have surely noticed by now, some adaptations of ancient sex techniques are sprinkled throughout this book. If you want to delay ejaculation, expand orgasm, and increase the intensity of an intimate encounter, you can do no better than turn to the old masters. In researching sex, I have been struck by how sexologists and sex therapists of the late twentieth century developed theories and techniques that are similar to the theories and techniques espoused and practiced by the sex experts of thousands of years ago.

Whether or not savvy modern lovers know the origins of the techniques they practice, they borrow from the ancients, from the great twentieth-century sex researchers, and from the prosex feminists who insisted men learn their way around the clitoris—and other sources.

If you want to go further into Tantra or Tao, this section will give you a taste of the real thing. The techniques are a bit more esoteric than the adaptations you've been learning in this book. Understanding the philosophy behind them is part of the lesson.

Everything sexual begins in the carnal old country, India. Just as we all came from the womb of an Eve in the African savanna, our sex lives came from the Hindu temples of India. Tantra is the root of ancient sex. The word is Sanskrit and loosely translated means "to weave" and "to extend."

In its pure form, Tantra is based on the belief that energy flows through the body in the same way that blood flows through the circulatory system. This energy runs through the body's "chakras," or energy centers, at the base of the spine, the genitals, the stomach, the throat, the forehead, and the crown of the head. According to Tantric philosophy, you can control how your energy travels that inner path and reach enlightenment.

Here's the good news: Sex can get you there.

Unlike most mystical paths, Tantra included sexuality as a doorway to ecstasy and enlightenment. Tantric sex "opens up the chakras"—which leads to spiritual enlightenment—by moving the energy up the body through these points into the top of the head, where that energy ultimately suffuses a sensation of oneness and ecstasy. Yes, that's a tough concept for the modern couple to wrap their brains, much less their legs, around.

TANTRIC SEX

Tantra was established five thousand years ago in India as a rebellion against the Brahmans, the Hindu priesthood, who preached sexual denial in the pursuit of spiritual enlightenment. (Imagine if Martin Luther had been a sex cult founder instead of a Protestant.) The Tantrics worshipped the god Shiva—who represents male energy—and his consort, the goddess Shakti—female energy—who they believed united the spiritual and the sexual, the male and the female energies. The Tantric tradition was carried to Tibet around the tenth century. Scattered underground cults were said to exist as far away as Athens and may have influenced some of the erotic traditions for prolonging pleasure and extending orgasm that exist in many cultures around the world, including Chinese, Greek, Native American, Polynesian, Egyptian, Scandinavian, and African.

However they came into being, those traditions include a variety of techniques unknown in Western culture. One ancient Polynesian sexual practice, for example, recommends an hour-long embrace of intercourse during which man and woman alternate periods of gentle movement with stillness to encourage a long and gentle orgasm, much like Karezza (page 165). The ancient Arabs practiced *Imsak*, the Arabic word for "retention," in which the man pulled out when he felt close to ejaculating and continued to stimulate the woman with his hands or mouth, until he was able to resume thrusting. That is exactly the theory behind the modern techniques for delaying his orgasm and increasing her arousal.

But the Arab lover would do this repeatedly, up to ten times per night, both to prolong his lover's pleasure by multiplying and extending her orgasms and to make his own orgasms stronger and longer by delaying them. In the Western world, men learned how to ejaculate as quickly as possible to avoid being caught masturbating. The veil of sin always hung over sexual expression. Women were given the messages that sex before marriage was especially bad for them because it would make them less desirable as wives—and that someday the prince would marry them and know how to make them come. Thanks to the glory that was the British Empire, these ideas about sex and morality were absorbed by other modern cultures, including India—the place where sacred sexuality was born.

Belatedly, we are learning from the ancients.

"Real talk"

"Tantra is about diving deeply into desire and pleasure," says Maya, who, with her husband, Bill, has been studying Tantric sex for two years. "Some of what you're told is discouraging, especially for Americans. Our first instructor in erotic massage said that you have to give each other a hundred massages to be really good at it. Please! Who wants to hear that?

"We were discouraged and might have quit. But Bill said, 'Let's take what we want from this. We'll keep going as long as we are learning and having fun. No pressure. We aren't kids in school who have to cram for the exam.'

"That is our philosophy. It works for us. We have learned a lot and we are better lovers, more deeply intimate with each other. When somebody tells us we aren't ready for the technique in the next section, we skip ahead and do it anyway. Often we have found that the technique is even better after we've progressed to where we were told we needed to be in the first place.

"But there are no bad or incorrect orgasms. We enjoy."

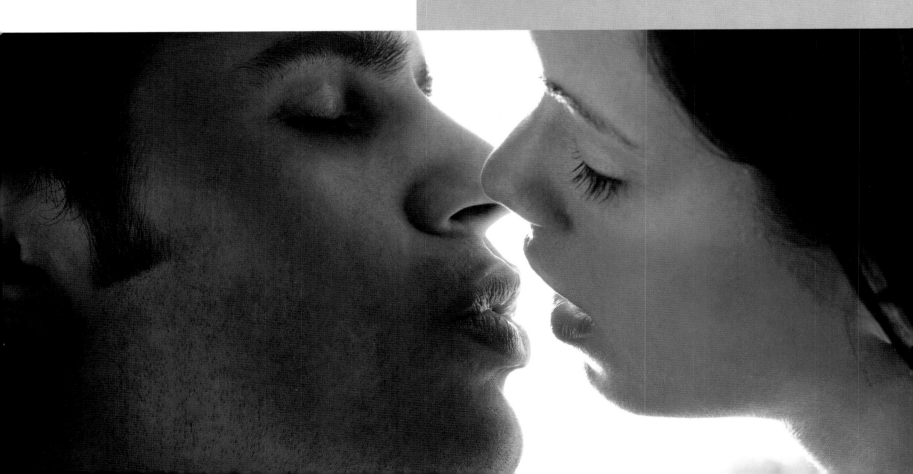

The Lessons of Tantra

Books about Tantra are inevitably wordy. Cutting through the verbiage to get to the lessons applicable to your love life is akin to cutting your way through kudzu (the vine that overtakes everything!) in the South.

The biggest difference between sex as you probably know it and Tantra is that Tantra lasts longer. While intercourse (not counting foreplay) is typically over in less than ten minutes, couples practicing Tantra can sustain an act of intercourse for up to an hour. Some claim longer records, but obviously there is no proof. (The rock star Sting admitted that he was only joking when he said that he, practicing Tantra, could make love for hours. The story was repeated in articles about him so often that he finally issued a denial.)

The lessons any couple can take away from Tantra:

■ Delay his orgasm.

■ Increase her arousal.

■ Intensify the intimate connection.

■ Increase orgasmic potential.

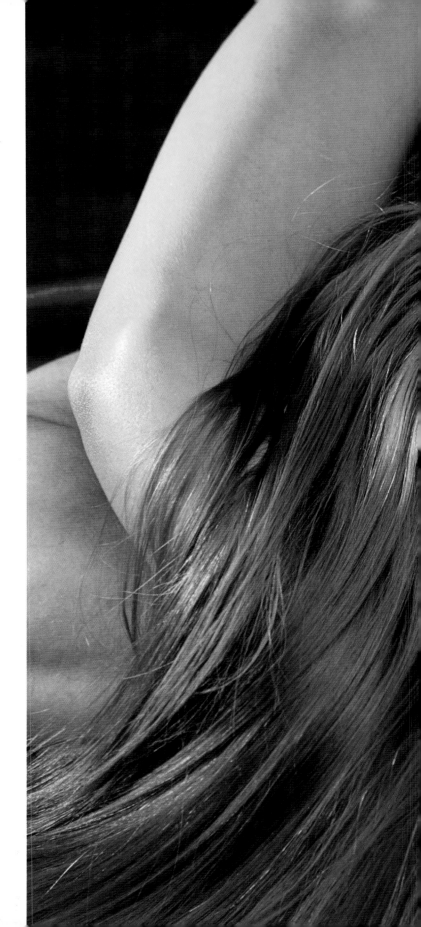

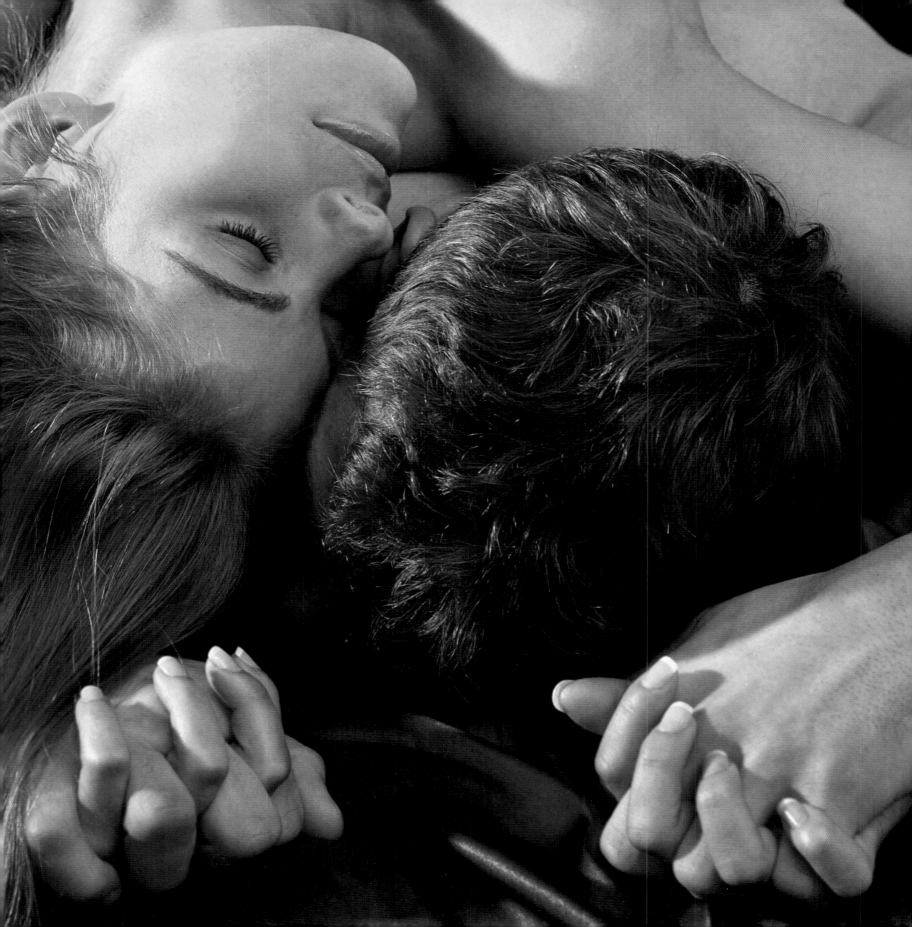

Can you practice Tantric sex?

Given the time commitment involved in reading the material, taking the classes, learning the positions and techniques, and putting it all into practice, Tantric sex is not for casual lovers nor for many time-pressured modern couples, either.

Margot Anand, the reigning international priestess of Tantra, warns readers in the introduction to her classic work, *The Art of Sexual Ecstasy*, that her book contains about fifty practice exercises—totaling seventy-five hours of activity—and that's just to get them started. The couple must purify their bodies, create a sacred space, learn how to breathe correctly, heal their inner wounds, overcome their inhibitions, and harmonize their "inner man and inner woman" before they get to anything we recognize as sex.

Lovers new to Tantra are discouraged by instructors from even attempting Riding the Wave of Bliss, a seven-step process to—one hopes—a big orgasmic conclusion.

Few couples will have both the time and the inclination to practice Tantric sex. But many couples will take away the basic lessons of Tantra and adapt some of the positions and techniques. The purists call that Tantra Lite, but Anand doesn't deride it.

Easy Tantra for modern lovers

The most accessible Tantra techniques are the Eye Lock, the Tantric Kiss, and the Yab-Yum position.

THE EYE LOCK

If you take nothing else away from Tantra, learn this technique. In holding your lover's gaze during foreplay, especially kissing, you deepen the intimate connection between the two of you to a degree you can't imagine before you try it. This is more than opening your eyes. You may feel naked and embarrassed at first; but do it.

Technique Tip

THE EYE LOCK

Look deeply into each other's eyes as you are caressing each other's bodies. Hold the look. Do this more than once. You probably won't realize how little you do look into each other's eyes during lovemaking until you practice the Eye Lock.

As you become more comfortable with locking eyes, concentrate on opening yourself up to your lover.

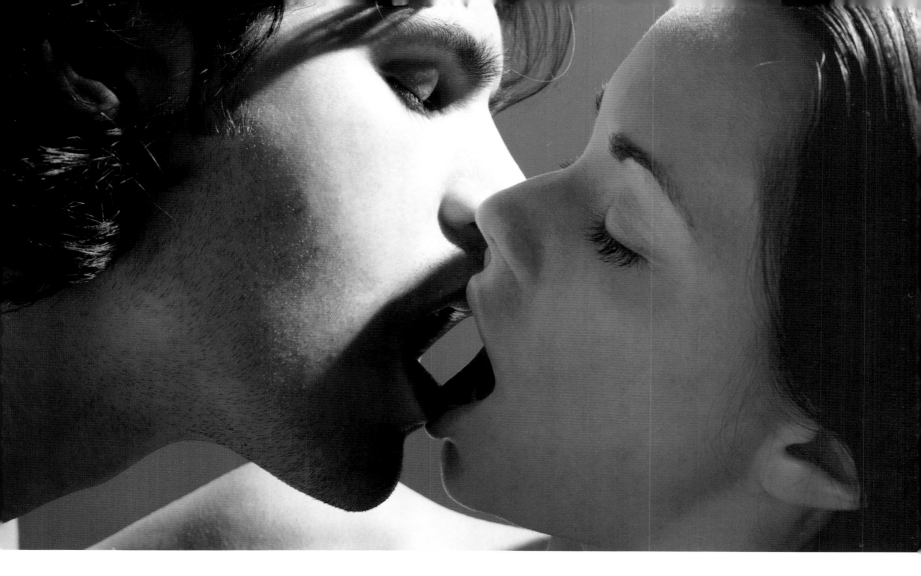

THE TANTRIC KISS

It's the ultimate soul mate kiss—and it's all about the breathing.

The concept: Sharing breath in your kiss is really a sharing of souls. Some Tantric guidebooks turn the kiss into an endurance contest. It's simple. You don't have to kiss longer than you feel inspired to. Just breathe into each other as you do it.

THE TANTRIC KISS

Sit on his lap and rock back and forth together for a minute to establish an intimate rhythm. Press your foreheads together for a minute or more. Play with each other's lips and tongues. Now bring your lips together in a real kiss. Inhale while he's exhaling and vice versa. As he breathes out, you are breathing his breath into your body. Feel it. As you exhale, you are giving yourself to your lover in your breath.

Now kiss and breathe into each other's mouths.

The Yab-Yum Position

Sit in the center of the bed (or floor) facing each other. Wrap your legs around each other so that she is "sitting" on his legs. Place your right hand at the back of your lover's neck, your left hand on his or her tailbone.

Each press your palm firmly at the base of the other's spine. Slide your hand up your lover's back to the base of his or her neck. Imagine that, as you slide your hand, you are channeling sexual energy up through your lover's body, warming him or her from genitals through heart, through head. Repeat the stroke over and over until you are both feeling very aroused.

Insert his penis into her vagina so that the shaft exerts as much indirect pressure as possible on her clitoris. Rock slowly together as you rub each other's backs and perform the Eye Lock.

After her orgasm, make love in other positions, varying the speed, thrust, and angle of thrusting to prolong his excitation phase as long as possible.

THE YAB-YUM

The Yab-Yum is definitely not a quickie position. Allow time for lovemaking. Light candles, burn incense, arrange fresh flowers in a vase on the bedside table, play soft music.

Lie in each other's arms. Stroke and caress and fondle each part of the other's body, except the genitals. Devote as much time to this luxurious state of foreplay as necessary to reach the point where you are aching to touch and be touched—in the genitals, of course.

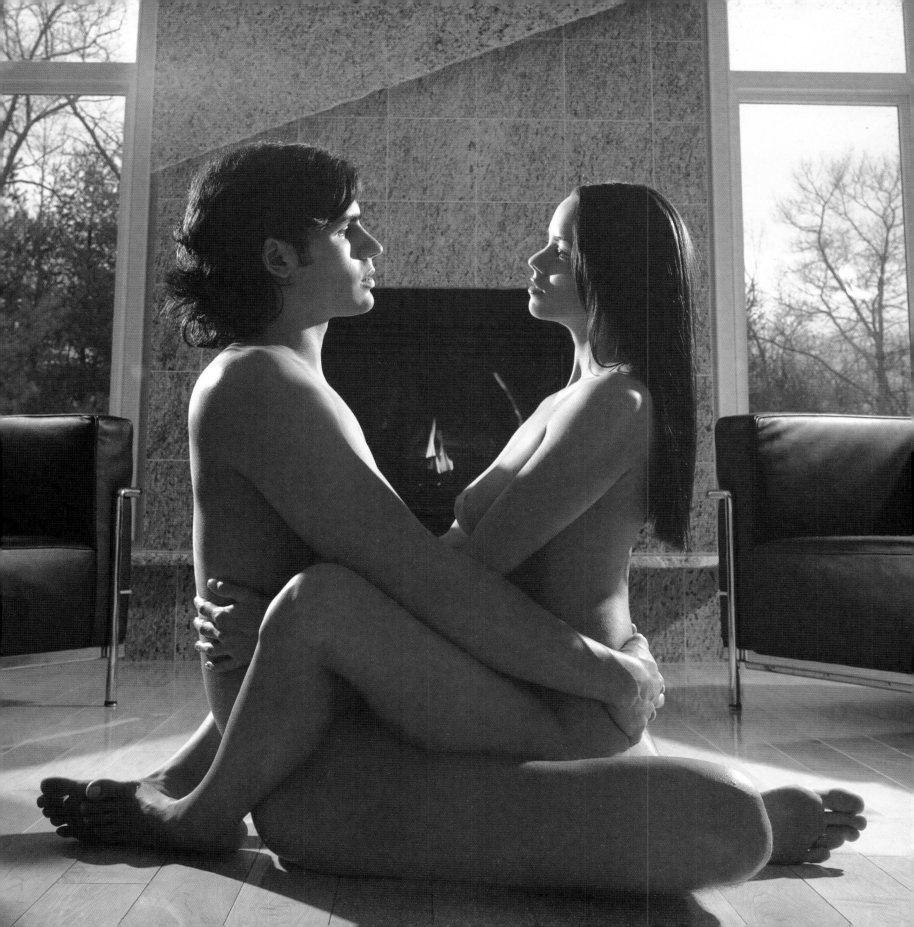

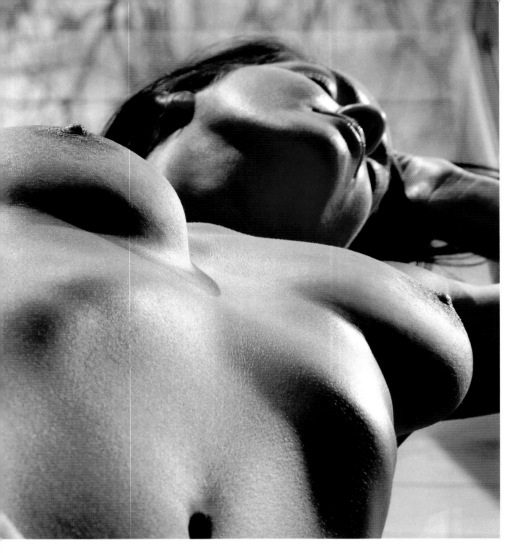

Deconstructing the Kama Sutra

The Kama Sutra, the most famous sex book in history, is a classic treatise on sex. It is adapted from the Kama Shastra—or "rules of love"—written by ancient Indian sages who based their philosophy of sex on teachings known as the Vedas, perhaps the world's oldest sacred text. The first version of the Kama Shastra is attributed in Hindu mythology to Nandi, Shiva's companion.

Fifteen hundred years ago, during India's golden period of the Gupta dynasty, Maharishi Vatsyayana, famous Indian sage and authority on sacred scriptures such as the Vedas, wrote the Kama Sutra, based on his translation and understanding of the Kama Shastra. Vatsyayana's Kama Sutra was recognized as the true text of the Kama Shastra and was clearly a unique work with universal appeal from the beginning. His bold treatment of sex as both science and art is brilliant—and certainly ahead of anything written on the subject in the Western world. And as he enumerates the scientific principles of lovemaking, he never fails to grasp the role that psychology plays in intimate behavior. A modest man, Vatsyayana claimed he only quoted and condensed the earlier work—and he refers to himself in the third person when he expresses an opinion.

"The Kama Sutra is not a pornographic work. First and foremost, it is a picture of the art of living for the civilized and refined citizen, combining in the sphere of love, eroticism and the pleasures of life."

— Alain Daniélou
Author and translator, whose *The Complete Kama Sutra* (1994) is regarded as the finest literary translation of that work

The Vedas state that the purpose of human life has four parts—*dharma* (duty), *artha* (wealth), *kama* (pleasure), and *moksha* (enlightenment of the soul). *Kama*, or sex, is indispensable. Not only can one be unhappy and unfulfilled without sex—one is also unable to reach enlightenment without it.

Kama Sutra describes sixty-four lovemaking practices, a set of erotic arts known as Panchali. A courtesan proficient in all sixty-four practices was known as a *ganika*, or sacred priestess of sex. Wealthy men, including royalty, compensated her for her favors and the enlightenment she helped them gain with generous offerings of money and precious gifts.

The Kama Sutra maintains that men and women are each divided into three categories: the man as rabbit, bull, and horse; the woman as dove, mare, and she-elephant. Each category has its own characteristics—and some of the women are described in unflattering terms. The rabbit is handsome, tender, and soft-spoken. The bull is stout and well-endowed with a large and shapely penis. The sturdy horse is long-faced but sexually passionate. Only the dove is very attractive. She is described as exceptionally beautiful, engaging, and soft-spoken, and her discharges are as fragrant as the blossoming lotus. The mare woman is slim, tall, and easily seduced—and she has a fishy aroma. But the she-elephant, a fat, gluttonous woman, awkward in demeanor, is the most highly sexed.

In the Kama Sutra, a harmonious sexual relationship depends upon a man and a woman's having compatible genitals. Otherwise their sexual and married life will prove disastrous. (Doesn't give the she-elephant a lot of options, does it?)

And if that happens_there are prescriptions for various Ayurvedic (traditional Indian medicine) recipes for those men and women whose physical or psychological problems interfere with their ability to have sexual intercourse. Sexology, psychology, medicine—and geography! In the Kama Sutra, one of the few ancient treatises referring to the geography of India, Vatsyayana says that women's sexuality is determined by climate.

It's a fascinating read.

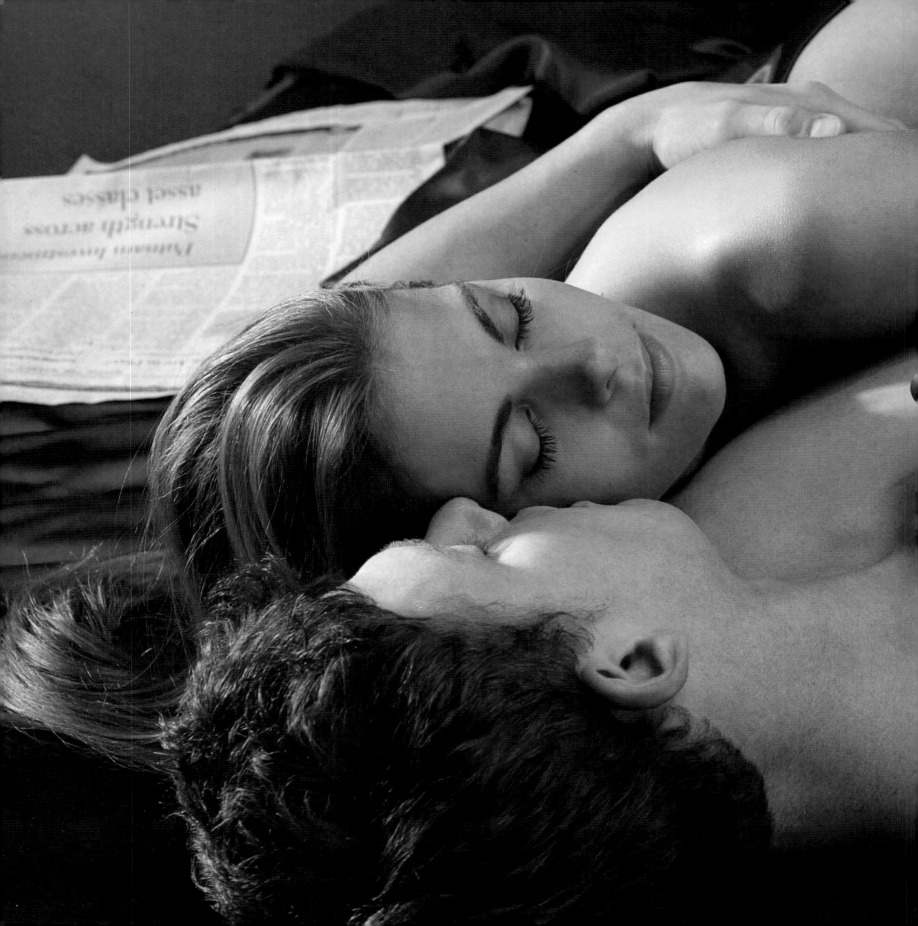

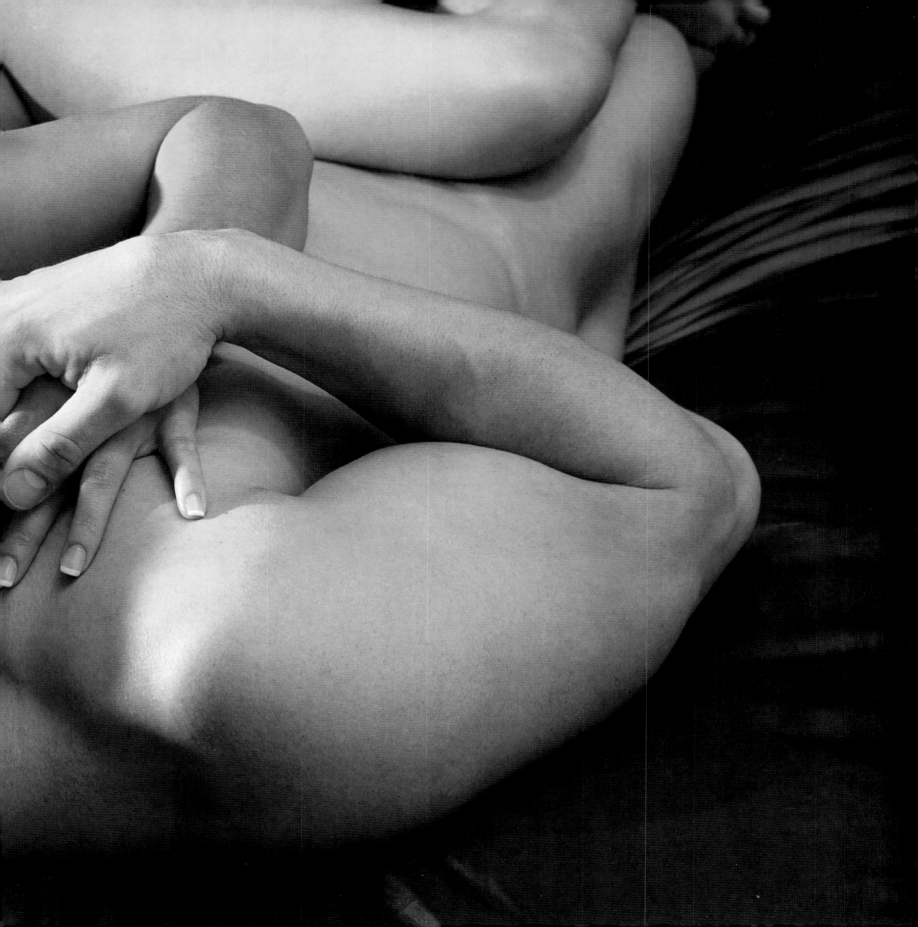

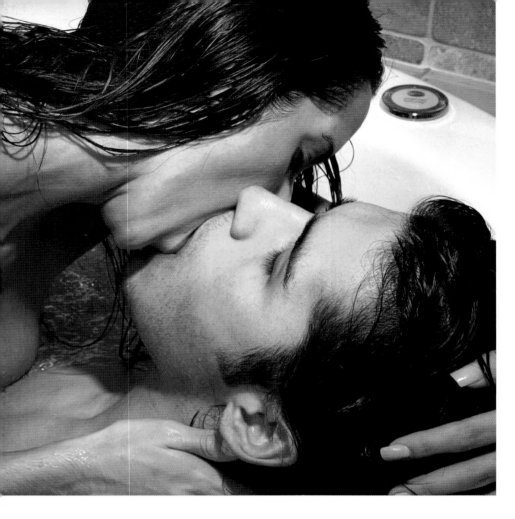

The Best of the Kama Sutra for Modern Lovers

Most versions of the Kama Sutra cut to the chase: the positions and the techniques.

The three areas of classic advice particularly relevant to couples today are kissing, embracing, and, of course, positions.

KISSING

The Kama Sutra has a good primer on the art of kissing—in other words, kissing the way women like it, long and sensuous. But there's something for the guys—and also for women when they're feeling more sizzling than romantic. Sometimes you like it soft, and sometimes you like it rough.

Biting, hard sucking, squeezing, and scratching are some of the love-play activities described in the world's first sex guide. There are detailed directions telling lovers how to leave different-shaped marks—which that we call "hickeys"—as a sign of sexual prowess on the man's part and passionate commitment on the woman's. In ancient India, both men and women grew one or more nails long specifically for the purpose of scratching their lovers.

While the Kama Sutra didn't instruct devotees in S/M, it did say that a woman's lips, bruised from kissing, were a badge of her desirability.

Here are my adaptations of the best Kama Sutra kissing techniques:

"Real talk"

"Tantric kissing and embracing are sensual," says Cherise, "and sensuality is the part missing from Western sex. We know how to do it hot, hard, and fast—because porn is our model for sexual contact. Tantra reminds you that there is a sensual, spiritual element to sexuality. You become aware of your partner's soul or essence or inner self, however you want to phrase it. You feel each other's souls in the kisses and touches. It heightens everything. Then when you move to hot, hard, fast sex, you are going there with someone you are actually touching."

TURNING THE KISS

According to the Kama Sutra, the position of the lovers' faces determines the type of kiss they are exchanging.

For example, the bent kiss is described this way: "When the heads of the two lovers are bent toward each other, and when so bent, kissing takes place, it is called the bent kiss." The bent kiss is also known as both the most popular and the gentlest of kisses.

You can change the energy by changing the direction of your faces.

To take the lead in making the kiss more personal, turn up your lover's face, by holding the chin or taking the face in both hands.

Increase the passion by taking both of your lover's lips between your own in the "clasping kiss." (According to the Kama Sutra, men with mustaches cannot kiss this way.)

And, finally, increase the intensity of the kiss and change it to "Fighting for the Tongue" by using the tip of your tongue on your lover's teeth, tongue, and palate.

EMBRACING

An embrace can be casual and affectionate—such as a hug exchanged between friends—or the intense prelude to intercourse. The Kama Sutra analyzes every degree of connection as the lovers move from the initial light touches to the full-body press. Here are my adaptations of the best embracing moves:

THE FOREHEAD KISS

In the "embrace of the forehead," one lover touches the mouth, the eyes, and the forehead of the other with his or her own forehead.

Don't laugh. Try it. Using your forehead to "kiss" your lover is a surprisingly intimate and affectionate move.

ESCALATING THE EMBRACE

A gentle, unexpected touch can be erotic or simply a display of affection.

Strictly speaking Kama Sutra, the "touching embrace" occurs when a man moves in front of or beside his woman and touches her body with his own. In the more practical version, it is a series of light touches over a period of an hour or more to your lover's hands, arms, shoulders, back—culminating in light brushes across her breast, his crotch.

These little touches create anticipation and expectation in your lover for the night ahead.

PRESSING THE EMBRACE

According to the book, in a pressing embrace a lover presses the other's body forcibly against a wall.

The full-body press—minus the element of force unless you're role-playing—is a sexy preforeplay move. Either hold your lover tightly against your body or lean him or her gently against a wall or a door in a theatrical flourish to your embrace.

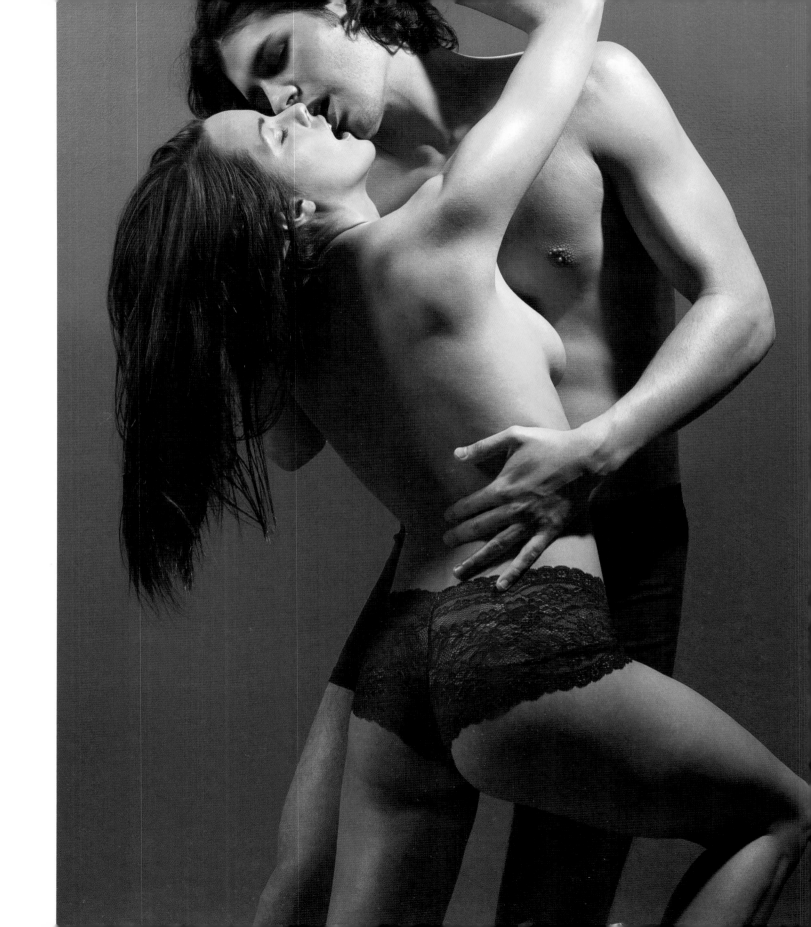

HER LEG WRAP

From the Kama Sutra: "When a woman, clinging to a man as a creeper twines around a tree, bends his head down to hers with the desire of kissing him and slightly makes the sound of sut sut, embraces him, and looks lovingly toward him, it is called the embrace of the twining creeper."

Never mind the "sut sut." Otherwise it is difficult to improve upon the classic embrace. Wrap one leg around his body, balance your weight against him, gently lower his face to yours—and kiss passionately. What man can resist?

THE FULL-BODY BACK SCRATCH

The "embrace of the Jaghana" won't appeal to many modern lovers. The man mounts his lover, scratches her with his nails as he bites, strikes, and finally kisses her. Don't go there.

But a full-body embrace combined with back-scratching can be deliciously seductive. On a sofa, bed, or carpeted floor, lie in each other's arms. Embrace fully. Take turns scratching each other's backs.

INTERCOURSE

Even people who have never seen a translation of the Kama Sutra associate the sacred text with intercourse positions—a dizzying array of them. Many, if not most, of the positions are not likely to be achieved by couples who aren't young, slim, fit, and very flexible. However, they can be adapted.

Use the positions of the Kama Sutra as inspiration, not dogma. Let the photos and drawings arouse you. Then figure out how they can work for you.

Here are my adaptations of some very hot Kama Sutra positions—designed for her maximum stimulation and his maximum endurance.

THE FROG ▶

Most couples will be able to maintain this position for only a few minutes. It requires strong thigh muscles in him—and, once again, a good PC muscle in her. Prepare for the Frog to collapse gracefully into a version of the missionary position by placing behind her a few pillows that will lift her buttocks higher when she falls. Or he can fall back and bring her on top of him in the female superior position.

Legs apart, he squats. With her legs placed over his, she sits on his lap. He maintains a gentle rocking motion, while she sits still, moving with her PC muscle around the shaft of his penis. As her excitement grows, she begins to rock gently in time with his movements.

And, depending upon their mood, they fall back in one direction or the other.

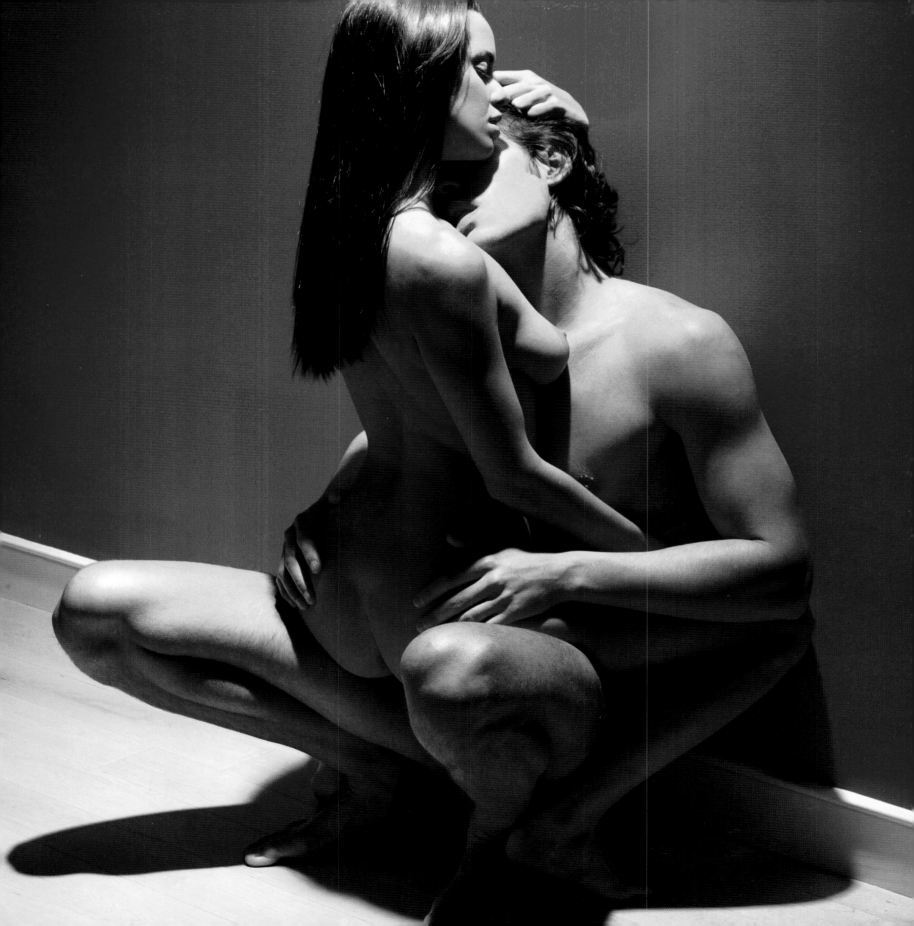

PLAYING AT THE EDGE

In many translations of the text, this position is called "Putting On the Sock." Go figure.

She lies on her back. He sits between her legs with his penis at the entrance to her vagina. He slowly caresses her vagina with his fingers until she is very wet. Then he gently inserts the head of his penis into her vagina. He stimulates her clitoris with his fingers as he strokes her vagina with the head of his penis.

When she is on the verge of orgasm, he thrusts deeply and rapidly—while continuing the clitoral stimulation if she needs that.

BUILDING A FIRE

In a variation of the previous position, she lies down and draws her knees to her torso. Her vagina is pushed forward. He will find that view exciting as he kneels before her.

His objective? Tease her to the point of madness by inserting and withdrawing his penis. (He will probably need to add clitoral stimulation, either with the head of his penis or with his fingers, to really drive her mad.)

Called "The Blacksmith's Posture," this position got its name because it imitates the blacksmith drawing the hot iron from the fire and plunging it back in again. Obviously she has a limited range of motion—and that helps maintain his erection longer.

Once she—and likely he—reaches the "mad" point, they will slip into a position more compatible with hard-driving sex.

THE CHARIOT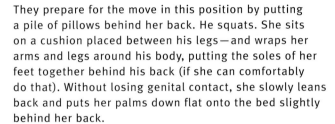

They prepare for the move in this position by putting a pile of pillows behind her back. He squats. She sits on a cushion placed between his legs—and wraps her arms and legs around his body, putting the soles of her feet together behind his back (if she can comfortably do that). Without losing genital contact, she slowly leans back and puts her palms down flat onto the bed slightly behind her back.

Now he stretches back, putting his palms onto the bed in the same way she has done. They rest their legs on the other's shoulders.

Movement is a slow and delicious balancing act. When things heat up, they can move to any position that facilitates orgasm.

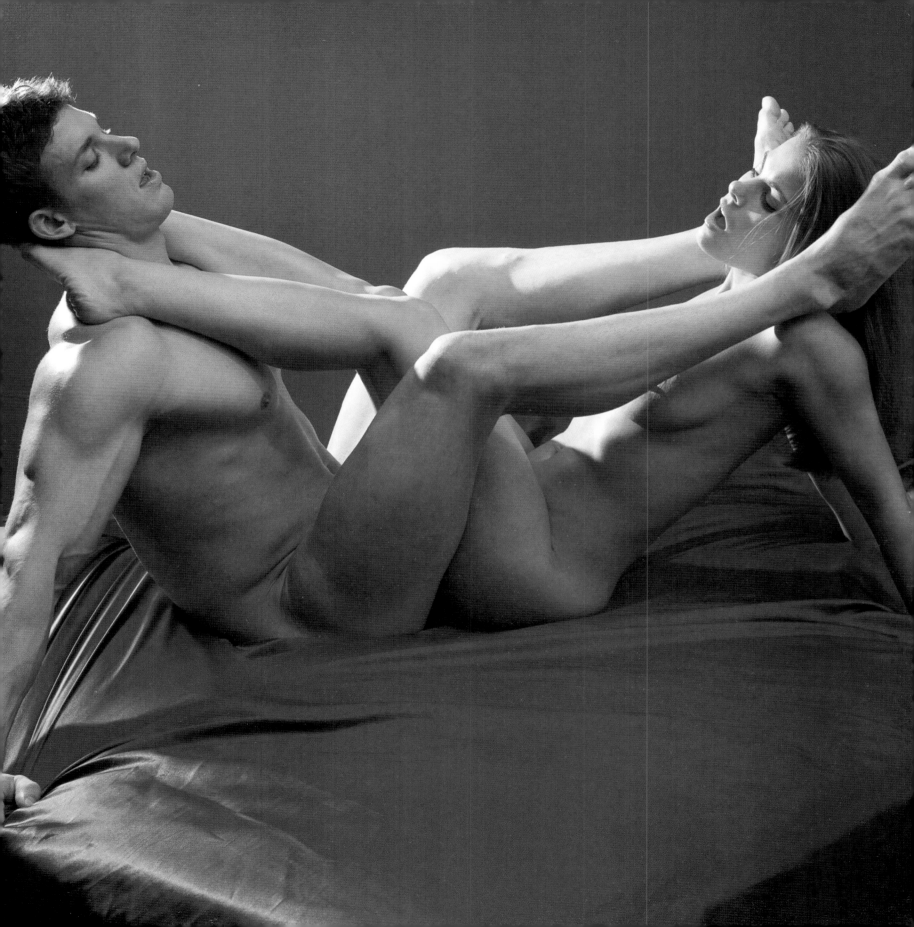

THE SLANTED WOMAN

She lies on her back. Again, he kneels in front of her, but this time at her feet. He raises her legs until only her head and shoulders remain on the bed or the floor. He moves closer to her vagina. After he enters her, she puts her legs around his head. (A graduated stack of pillows will make this a doable position for more couples.)

Called "The Ostrich's Tail" because her raised legs give the impression of being spread out—like an ostrich's tail—this technique works for both of them. She gets G-spot stimulation. He can (as always) stimulate her clitoris. And the bonus: The position helps him last longer.

THE WHEELBARROW ▶

This is a great position for stimulating the G-spot! But it also requires flexibility and careful positioning.

She starts by standing, and then bends over with her head and arms resting on the floor (or bed or chair). He stands behind her and grabs one of her ankles. She should keep one knee slightly bent as she shifts her weight to the leg that's still on the floor.

He lifts both feet to rest near his hips, and then moves forward to engage her. She then wraps her legs around his back, while he holds on to her lower back or buttocks as he moves in and out of her.

When the position becomes uncomfortable for her—or they want more vigorous thrusting—they shift into one of the basic positions.

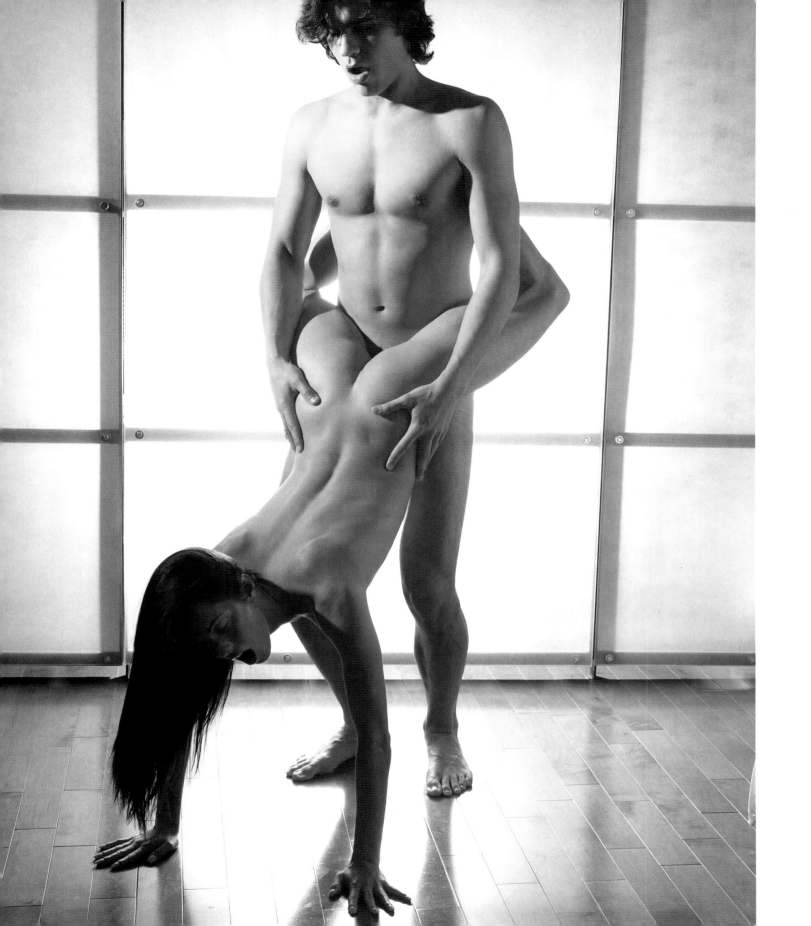

OPENING HEAVEN'S GATES

A slight variation on the Kama Sutra's "Yawning Position," this one also puts the woman on her back. She raises and spreads her legs as wide as she comfortably can. He enters her vagina.

In addition to giving the benefits of the others, this one really allows the lovers to be intimate. They can gaze into each other's eyes—and, in fact, practice the Eye Lock (see page 176). She can caress her breasts, adding to his visual stimulation.

Use pillows beneath her back or buttocks to achieve the angle most beneficial for her orgasm.

THE SULTAN ▶

He's tired—or she wants to pamper him. She sits up, her back against pillows or a padded headboard. With his legs wrapped around her body, soles touching behind her back, he sits inside her legs. They wrap their arms around each other and kiss and caress in this embrace.

Once he has a firm erection, he lies back on the bed with his legs up, ankles resting on her shoulders. She guides him inside her, and she controls the thrusting. Her hands are free to stimulate her own clitoris—and massage his perineum.

Some other positions in other parts of this book have been adapted from the Kama Sutra, most notably the X position on (page 125). Be creative. Make your own adjustments to these and other positions.

The goals are always: Increase stimulation to her clitoris and G-spot—thus increasing her arousal—while helping him delay ejaculation.

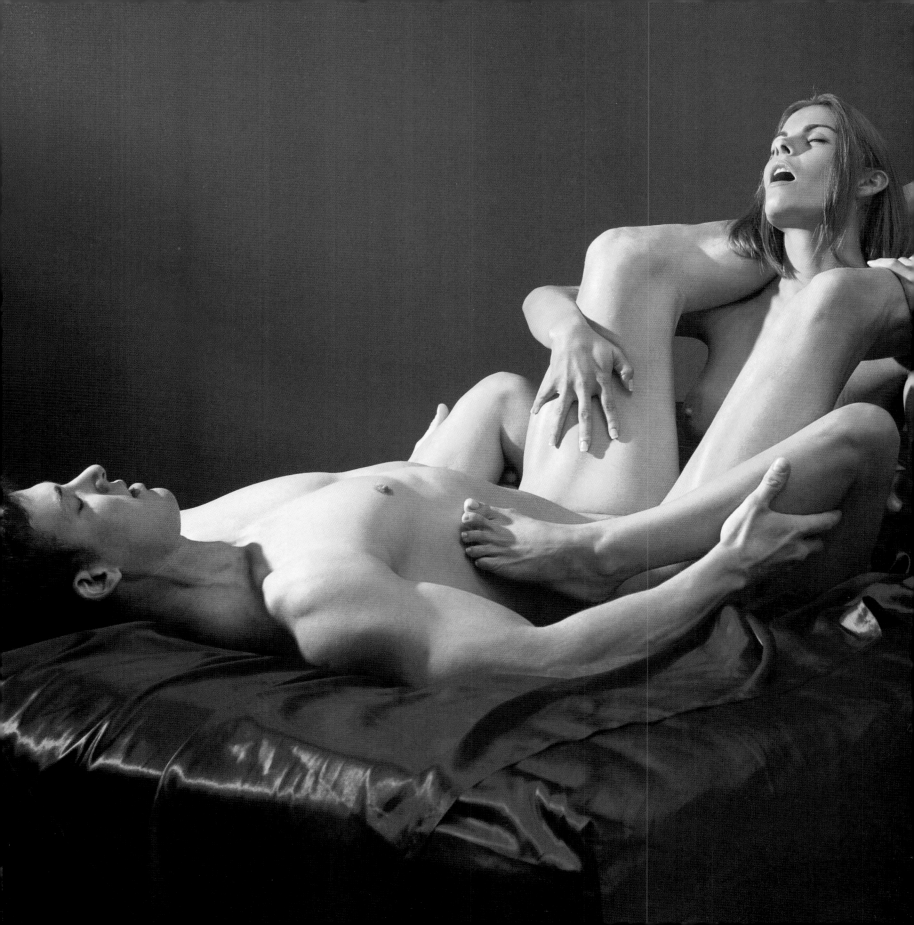

Taoist Sex

Tantra's lesser-known cousin, Taoist sex began two thousand years ago in China. Chinese physicians studied sex and decided that lovemaking was necessary to the physical, mental, and spiritual well-being of men and women. And then, of course, they had to tell men and women how to have that sex.

According to Taoist belief, energy is the source of all life. To maintain a dynamic balance of health, humans—relatively minor players in the grand scheme of nature—must be in harmony with energy. The Tao purports to show people how to do that by balancing the yin (feminine energy) and the yang (masculine energy). Lovemaking plays a vital role in the balancing act, because the most accessible energy is sexual attraction.

Neither a religion with secret rituals and deities nor a path to salvation, the Tao is the infinite force of nature, the path of the heart—or simply "the way." Sex is not sacred but a form of medicine—a healing force. The Tao is a sex-positive approach that helps better integrate sexuality with spiritual growth, with these primary goals for lovers:

- Sustaining male erection—and delaying ejaculation.

- Redirecting sexual energy in both men and women through the body into higher regions of the heart and the brain.

- Exchanging their energy with each other.

THE TAOIST EJACULATION TEACHINGS

Many in the Western world believe that Taoists strive to abstain from ejaculation altogether. That's not true. Male semen is regarded as a vital essence. Taoism does teach extended ejaculation control, but men are allowed to ejaculate—ideally two or three times in ten lovemaking episodes.

The belief that male orgasm and ejaculation are not the same thing comes from the Tao. The philosophy isn't designed to punish him but to teach him how to enjoy the high pleasure of orgasm without always experiencing ejaculation. Ejaculatory control is thought to conserve his energy, improve his lovemaking, stimulate his immune system, and make him love his partner even more.

Yes, that sounds like a lot to expect from holding back.

The following techniques have been adapted from Taoist teachings—to increase time spent on foreplay, stimulate and increase her arousal, delay his ejaculation, and intensify the intimate bond. Worthy goals—and it's always fun to aim for them.

Technique Tip

THE FOREPLAY ACCORDING TO TAO

She lies on her back with legs outstretched, slightly apart. He places his palm on her pelvic bone with three fingers curving over the clitoris and the vagina. (No insertion.)

He presses her for three to five seconds.

She pushes her pelvis against his curved hand, tightening the PC muscle and the muscles of her inner thighs as she breathes deeply and rhythmically.

Over the next three to five seconds, he lightens the pressure on her pelvis.

Now she pulls her pelvis back and releases the PC and inner thigh muscles—and breathes out.

Then repeat for several minutes.

He performs cunnilingus while stimulating her nipples with his fingers.

The foreplay should last at least twenty minutes.

"Ladies first, gentlemen. . . . Why?

Direct your attention to Lorena Bobbitt, who, when questioned

by police as to why she cut off her husband's penis, responded,

'He always has an orgasm and doesn't wait for me. It's unfair.'"

— Ian Kerner, Ph.D.
Clinical sexologist and author of
*She Comes First: The Thinking Man's
Guide to Pleasuring a Woman*

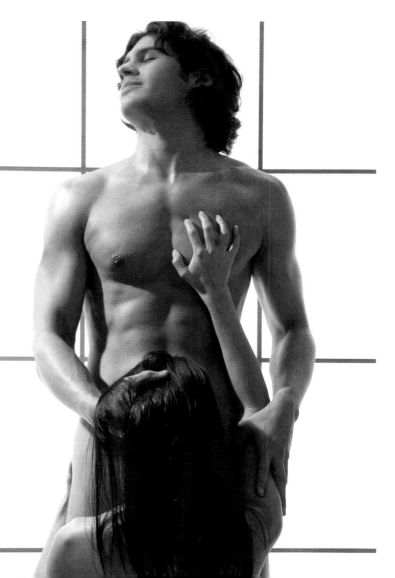

Her Tao Orgasm

In Tao, she comes first. That is also a modern Western viewpoint popularized during the Sexual Revolution and the Women's Movement of the '60s and '70s. Men began giving women the "first" orgasm via cunnilingus because women finally told them that two minutes of intercourse wasn't getting them there.

Technique Tip

THE TAO COMING

She can reach orgasm only in a face-to-face position—with legs outstretched, never bent.

When her orgasm is near, she firmly presses her entire body against his, rapidly pushing and pulling her pelvis.

His job: Don't breathe too hard and "receive steadily" her pelvic pushing while maintaining his deep penetration. He presses all his weight against her in "gentle movement."

They repeat "receiving her pelvic thrust" and his gentle movement alternately—at the rate of twice per second.

This has clearly been the inspiration for the CAT position (page 99). But here is where East and West part: When she reaches orgasm, he continues penetration and gentle movement—without ejaculating.

HIS TAO EJACULATORY CONTROL

He comes—maybe.

If he ejaculates within five minutes of penetration—
which most men do—he has failed. A good lover by
Taoist definition can sustain intercourse for
a minimum of twenty minutes—and preferably forty-five
minutes. Why so long? Women need at least twenty
minutes of intercourse (after thirty minutes of foreplay)
to reach orgasm—and, again, she comes first. (And she
comes with no hands.)

Before attempting the following technique, practice
Kegels (page 36) until your PC muscle is strong—and then
perfect the Big Draw (page 147) and the Three-Finger
Draw (page 147).

Technique Tip

THE TAO LONG WAY

1. Begin having intercourse with shallow penetration
   and slow thrusting.

   Contract the PC and abdominal muscles while slowly
   breathing air into the chest until you feel it expanding.
   Do this for seven to nine seconds. Now hold your breath
   and keep your muscles tight for another seven to nine
   seconds. Finally, still keeping the abdomen and the
   PC muscle contracted, breathe out for seven to nine
   seconds. Relax your muscles.

2. Penetrate more deeply now and thrust more vigorously.

   Then pause at the deepest point of insertion. Contract and
   relax the PC muscle as quickly as possible nine times.

3. Go back to shallow penetration and slow thrusting and
   repeat steps one and two.

4. Now repeat steps one and two again, but this time instead
   of finishing step one with relaxing muscles, add the nine
   rapid contractions of the PC muscle. In other words, both
   steps one and two end with nine rapid PC contractions.

   By now you've been having intercourse for at least fifteen
   minutes and possibly twenty.

   Keep repeating step four. If you feel that ejaculation
   is imminent, withdraw. Give your partner oral or manual
   stimulation for a few minutes. Then begin again.

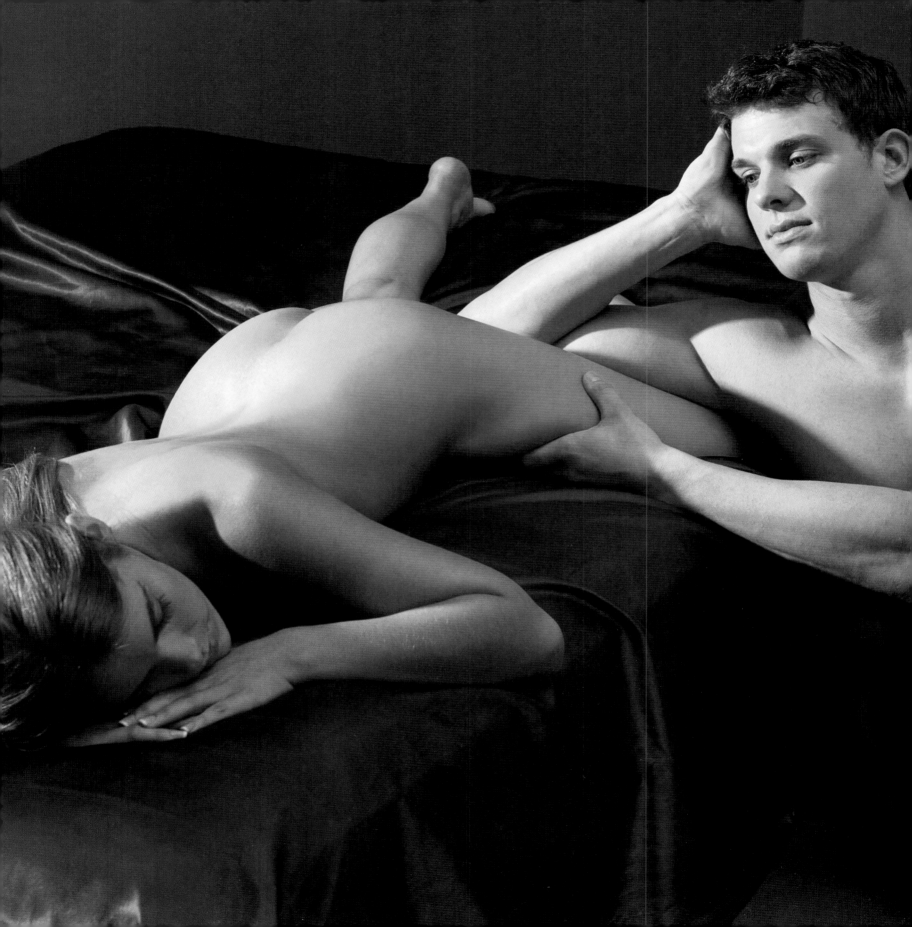

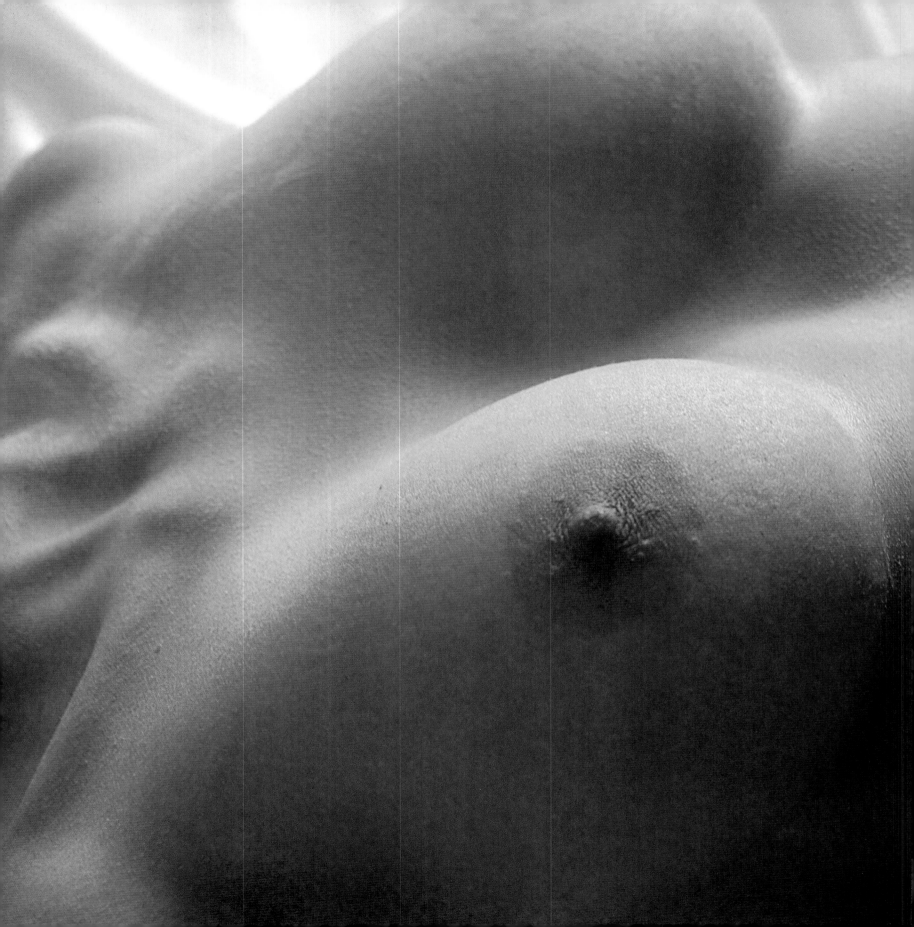

SEX TOYS
AND SEX GAMES

7

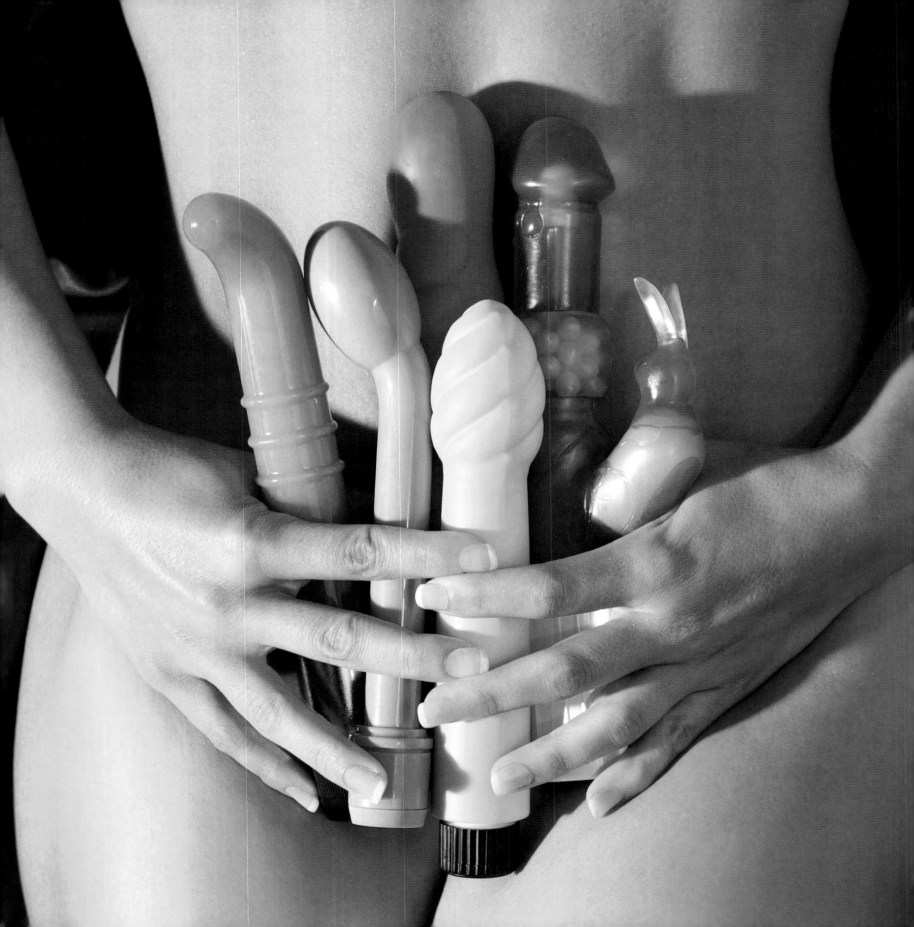

SEX TOYS

———

"It's rumored that Cleopatra kept a container,

perhaps a hard-shelled gourd, filled with live bees

for use as a primitive vibrator."

— Karen Eckhaus
Associate curator at The Museum of Sex
in New York City

Human beings have been fashioning phallic-shaped objects since prehistoric times, but the ancient Greeks are credited with first using them for sexual enhancement. Sex toys were very popular in Japan thousands of years ago. Early Japanese sex manuals illustrate a bewildering array of devices for use in masturbation and lovemaking. The classic ben-wa balls were introduced in that country. Lonely geishas and courtesans—who were thought to "need" more sexual satisfaction than wives—used them when their lovers were not around. The balls, inserted into the vagina, generated little waves of pleasure as the woman rocked in a chair or a swing.

VIBRATORS

Then shortly after the turn of the twentieth century in America, small battery-operated vibrators were available to doctors who prescribed them for their female patients suffering from "hysteria." Genital massage—believe it or not—was the standard treatment for female hysteria among enlightened doctors. The objective was to induce "hysterical paroxysm"—or orgasm—until the lady was cured.

By the 1920s vibrators were marketed as "massagers" to the general public. By the 1960s "female hysteria" had been debunked by the medical establishment—and vibrators were touted as the cure for the inorgasmic woman. She was warned, however, that she might grow so dependent on the vibrator that she wouldn't be able to have an orgasm without one.

"Vibrators are celebrated. They have a status of their own.

It's like a rock 'n' roll T-shirt. If you have a vibrator, it says you're

cool and hip. Women feel much more entitled to having great sex lives."

— Rachel Venning
Cofounder of Toys in Babeland

Most experts agree that that's not true. But a vibrator enthusiast may have to turn off the switch for a while.

Twenty years ago, in our modern world "sex toys" was a category that consisted largely of vibrators. A lot of women owned one, but they weren't as commonplace—or as high-tech—as they are now. Sex toy stores were typically purveyors of a limited style range of vibrators, large dildos in lurid colors, and very tacky crotchless panties. Toy stores aimed at women, Internet shopping, and sex toy parties have since made it possible for more women, especially those living outside major urban areas, to have their own high-quality toys. Cable shows such as *Sex and the City* made sex toy ownership desirable.

The two biggest and best sex toy stores for women are Good Vibrations, headquartered in San Francisco, and Toys in Babeland, which got its start in Seattle. Both have Web sites that provide a lot of useful information on sex techniques and practices, as well as a place to shop. And there's probably a Pleasure Chest store in your local mall.

Today's Best

By far the largest category—and best selling—of sex toys are vibrators. According to Venning, vibrators are more than 40 percent of Babeland's sales. A vibrator is also your indispensable toy because it can reliably accelerate arousal and induce orgasm. Though women buy and use most of them, they're not for women only. And one of the classics isn't even limited to genital use.

Here are the top six vibrators. And why stop with one?

The Hitachi Magic Wand

This large multiuse electric vibrator can be purchased next to the blow-dryers in drugstores and in the small-appliance section of department stores—as well as in sex toy shops. It's great for massaging back and shoulders. You can use it in couple play, for example, by placing it between your bodies in an intercourse position.

But its intensity may be too much for direct genital contact. Try leaving your panties on rather than starting on bare skin.

BEST FOR: women who have difficulty reaching orgasm; menopausal women who may need more stimulation to reach orgasm; any woman who wants an orgasm *now!*

The Pocket Rocket

This tiny vibrator looks like a fat tube of lipstick. But don't let its petite size fool you. The Pocket Rocket delivers on the promise inherent in its name. You can use it directly on your vulva and probably on your clitoris, too.

BEST FOR: traveling; stimulating his perineum.

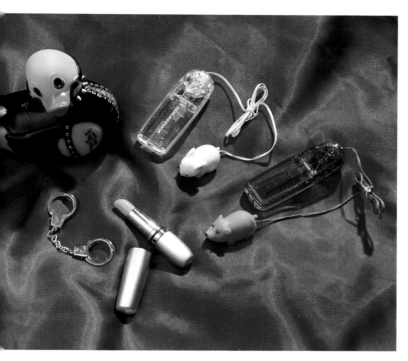

Right: Fortunately, vibrators have come a long way. Yesterday's frighteningly low-tech models have been replaced by more sleek, stylish, and discreet options (above), allowing women to achieve quick and powerful orgasms without the fear of the whole neighborhood overhearing—or electrocution, for that matter.

The Rabbit

Made famous by its popularity with the characters in *Sex and the City*, The Rabbit (and its dual-action clones) stimulates multiple areas of your vulva, vagina, and clitoris—all at once. You insert the shaft, which twirls and stimulates your G-spot while the "pearls" embedded in the base of the shaft stimulate your lower vagina. While all this is going on, the little rabbit attached to the shaft stimulates your clitoris with its ears.

BEST FOR: the adventurous woman who wants to experience an intense orgasm.

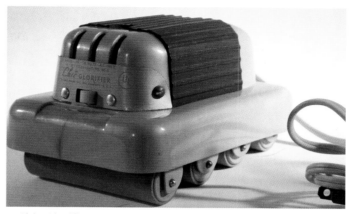

1. Chic Glorifier

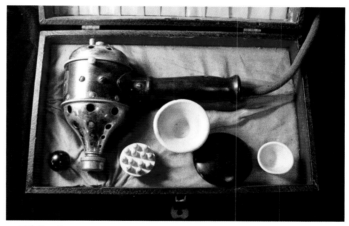

2. White Cross

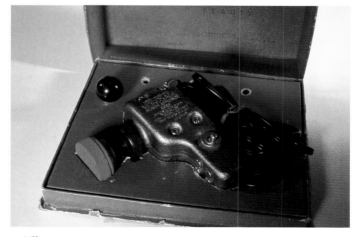

3. Vibrosage

The Talking Head Vibrator

The Talking Head tells women what they want to hear: You're beautiful, sexy, and desired.

Made of stunning blue-and-purple silicone, it has the same rotating pearls in the center of the shaft that other rabbits have—and the ears for clitoral stimulation. But Talking Head is no ordinary vibrator. It has a computer chip inside that produces CD-quality sound to let you customize and maximize your masturbation experience.

Do you want a French lover, an Italian, an African-American, a Latino—or another?

Put in the computerized chip and he will help you come.

BEST FOR: any woman who has ever wished her vibrator could talk.

The Strap-On Vibrator

You won't have trouble reaching orgasm during intercourse if you wear this small vibrator held in place against your clitoris by pretty straps. Not as powerful as its predecessors on this list, it will give you just enough extra stimulation to get you there. It is unobtrusive—and he may enjoy the mild sensations, too.

BEST FOR: intercourse.

The Natural Contours Vibrator

Designed by adult-filmmaker Candida Royalle, the Natural Contours Vibrator was created to fit the natural curve of your vulva. Gentle vibrations emanate from this sleek contemporary toy. If you want something free from phallic connotations, this is it.

BEST FOR: the woman new to sex toys.

The Basic Female Masturbation Technique

Most women reach orgasm with the vibrator by pressing it against their clitoris—often protected by silky panties—not via vaginal penetration. Experiment by varying the pressure and speed as you move the vibrator over your vulva, labia, and clitoris and surrounding tissue. If the vibration is too intense even at low speed for direct clitoral contact, move it to the side. Play with prolonging the excitation phase by moving the vibrator back and forth, from hot spot to not. Tease yourself to a stronger orgasm.

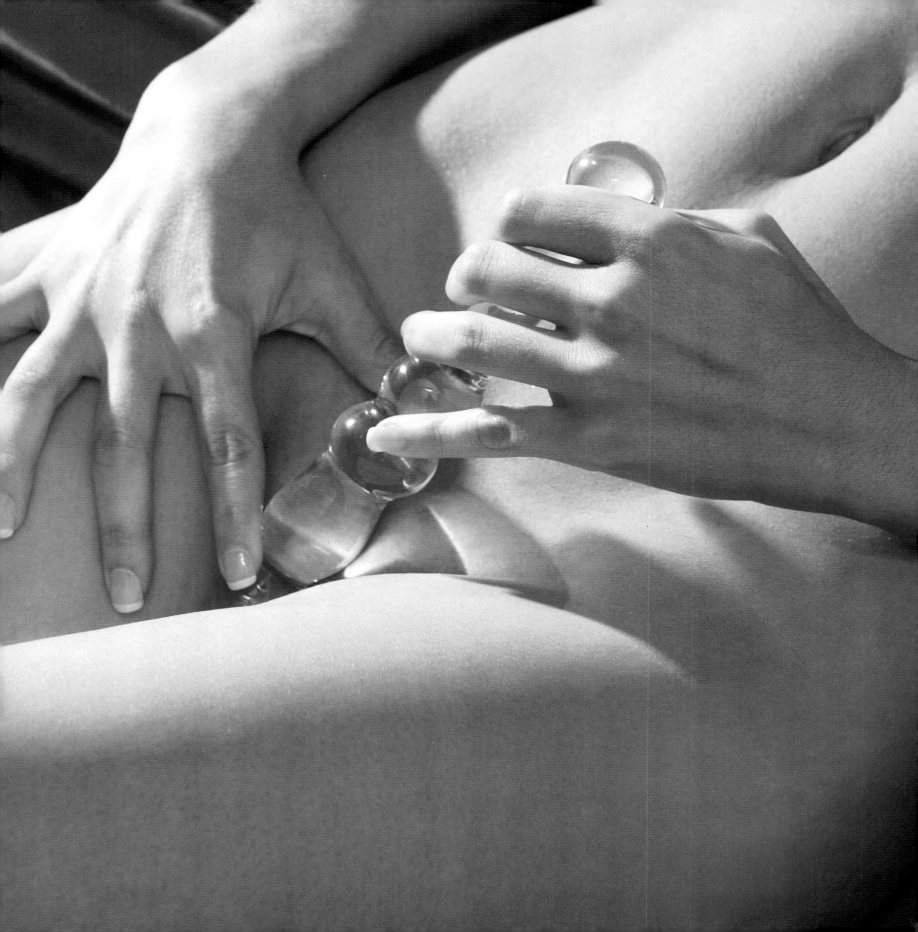

The Basic Male Masturbation Technique

Start on low speed. Run the vibrator along the shaft of the penis, then press it against the base, the scrotum, and the perineum. Experiment with higher speeds and firmer pressures. You can have a stronger orgasm by resisting the urge to grasp your penis and perform manual masturbation. Used correctly, the vibrator takes longer.

And that can be a good thing for both of you.

HIS VIBRATOR PLAY

Yes, he can play with a vibrator, too.

Typically men use vibrators on their partners only during couple sex play. Or, if you or his past partners are adventurous, he may have experienced the pleasurable sensations of her vibrator used on him. Some men are reluctant to admit how good it feels.

Technique Tip

THE VIBRATING COCK RING

The silicone ring attached to a vibrating torpedo and battery pack looks a bit strange. But you will love the way it feels. Place the stretchy cock ring around the base of your penis with the attached torpedo turned down to stimulate your perineum—or up during intercourse to stimulate her clitoris. Either way, you will feel the vibrations around the base of your penis.

Now turn it on.

"Real talk"

William says, "I was, as my girlfriend put it, 'squeam-ish' about having a vibrator used on me. I thought it was 'gay' or something. She said, 'Hey, it's motion. That's not gay or straight. See how it feels.' She had this little contour vibrator strapped on the back of her hand. She took my penis in that hand and I thought, Hey, this is good, this is really good."

COUPLE VIBRATOR PLAY

Here are six ways that couples can incorporate vibrators into their lovemaking:

1. TAKE TURNS massaging each other with the vibrator. Move down the body to the genitals, move away and back again, using the vibrator to tease as you would use your mouth or hands. Because it has a long handle and also works well as a body massager, the Hitachi Magic Wand is the one to use here.

2. USE THE VIBRATOR to vary stimulation while caressing your lover's genitals. A woman can hold the vibrator against the back of her hand that is cupping her partner's scrotum or holding his penis. A man can hold the vibrator against the back of his hand as he strokes her labia and the sides of her clitoris.

3. STIMULATE HIS (OR HER) perineum with a small vibrator, such as the Pocket Rocket, during oral or manual lovemaking.

4. USE THE G-SPOT VIBRATOR or a G-spot attachment to a multipurpose vibrator to stimulate her vagina during intercourse.

5. SHE CAN USE AN ANAL VIBRATOR on him while she performs fellatio or fondles his genitals. He can use an anal vibrator on her while he performs cunnilingus or manually stimulates her clitoris. Select a modest size and start with a low speed. Use lubrication and proceed slowly until your lover indicates a desire for more.

6. INSERT A WAND-SHAPED VIBRATOR between your bodies during intercourse. He will feel indirect vibrations throughout his penis inside her vagina as she is getting clitoral stimulation.

Dildos

Dildos are shaped like the penis. Unlike vibrators, they have no action component. They have probably been around since women figured out the connection between the excitement of being penetrated and the male organ. In ancient times, women used everything from smooth stones to vegetables such as long-necked squashes and cucumbers to stimulate themselves. You're lucky because you can select one from a wide array of colorful vibrators at your local sex toy shop.

Why bother when they don't vibrate?

Some women like to control the speed and motion of the thrusting. Using a dildo seems more like intercourse to them. They select dildos made of lifelike materials—and in sizes of actual penises. Huge dildos are more for show than for insertion. (If you want to play with one, use it to stroke your vulva, labia, and clitoris.)

STRAP-ON DILDOS

The unexpected success of the video series *Bend Over, Boyfriend* has widened the market for strap-on dildos, once a toy purchased primarily by lesbians, not straight women. Some men do enjoy anal penetration and some women are willing to oblige them. And other women say to their men, "If you want me to receive anal sex, you give that position a try for a change."

THE HARNESS STYLES

You can, of course, manually use a dildo to penetrate his anus, but a harness frees your hands for other pursuits—and gives you a new thrill, thrusting. If you don't own a dildo, you might want to buy a *strap-on kit* containing the dildo and a harness. That's a good option for beginners—and the woman who likes her dildo and harness color-coordinated. A bonus: The kit will come equipped with instructions, such as use a lot of lube.

Prepare him to receive anal sex in the same way he prepares you. Make sure he is aroused and well lubricated before you penetrate his anus. Insert the dildo slowly. Let him direct the depth of penetration and speed of thrusting.

The *basic harness* straps the dildo onto your body via adjustable straps around the waist and thighs. A *two-strap harness* has two leg straps that wrap around the thighs and attach to a slim waistband. A sexier option is the *G-string harness*. It looks like a leather thong with a single strap running up the center of the butt, attaching to a slim waistband.

The ultimate in strap-on pleasure is the *vibrating harness*. Two little vibrating pads are attached to the harness, one next to her clitoris, the other located where the dildo comes out of the harness. Hers and his.

Nipple Clamps

This is not a "woman only" toy. Men have nipples, too. Some men enjoy having their nipples tweaked, squeezed, pinched, licked, sucked, and bitten more than women do. In general, men prefer a firmer touch on their nipples and genitals than women do—though a lot of women like having their nipples and breasts handled roughly in the heat of passion, especially just before their menstrual period. (If you're going to experiment with S/M, that is the time to start.)

A woman may like nipple-clamp play. A man may love it.

If you've never seen a nipple clamp, you may be imagining some wicked device—or wooden clothespins like the ones used in very old porn flicks. Nipple clamps come in assorted styles. They keep the same kind of pressure on your lover's nipples that you would exert in pinching them. The bonus? Your hands are free to play elsewhere.

You can browse the nipple-clamp selection online at Babeland or Good Vibrations—or in your local sex toy shop.

Varieties include:

Tweezer clamps the best choice for beginners, are the most comfortable and look the least like something you'd see lying around the warden's office in a prison camp. The tension can be adjusted by sliding a small ring closer to or farther away from the nipple. Narrow, plastic-covered, curved wire ends close around the base of the nipples, leaving the tips standing proudly up.

Clover clamps are big and sturdy—and would be intimidating to the novice. The clamp's body has four open sections between articulated arms. The force is not adjustable and is relatively hard. Gripper pads, consisting of mini rubber disks with bumps, keep the clamps firmly in place without abrading the skin. Tugging on the chain momentarily tightens the pressure.

Kitty clamps are "alligator-type" clamps with an adjusting screw limiting how tightly they can be fastened—with attached cylindrical weights. (Ouch!) Turn the control dial on and the clamps hum, strumming the captive nipples. Rotate it up a notch or two and the clamps buzz like a vibrator and make the nipples dance. This is not a beginner's toy.

Technique Tip

CLAMPING THE NIPPLE

Prepare your lover. Make sure his or her nipples are erect. Suck, lick, and squeeze to get them there. Test the pressure by fastening the clamp to the web of skin between your lover's thumb and index finger.

Watch the clock. A clamp constricts (and possibly halts) the flow of blood to the clamped nipple and surrounding tissue. Don't leave the clamps on for more than ten to fifteen minutes at a time.

Start by clamping as much flesh as possible. Experiment over time by gradually clamping less flesh. The less you clamp, the more concentrated the pressure and the more intense the sensations. Never clip only the very end of the nipple. Not only will the sensation be too intense, you risk tearing flesh.

Once the clamps are firmly attached, you can tease your lover's nipples with your tongue or feathers. If the clamps are part of a master/slave game, you can make him or her get down on all fours—or attach the chain connecting the clamps to a slave collar. If your lover is into a little more pain, briefly hang light weights from the clamps as he or she is in the down-on-all-fours position.

Remember: The longer they're on, the more they hurt coming off. When the blood rushes back to the nipple, it hurts. Everybody has his or her own response to stimulation. Some like it light, some heavy. Get it wrong and the play becomes torture—definitely not sexy.

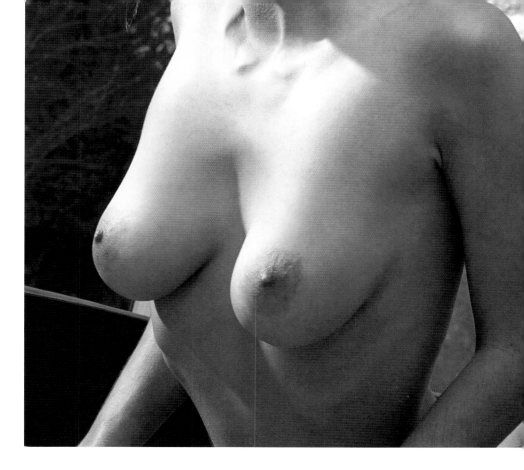

"Real talk"

"Inspired by a porn flick, my husband and I decided to try the strap-on," says Holly. "I am a fairly demure woman. When I saw the thing, I balked. He had a moment of regret, too. We drank some wine and said, 'Oh, what the hell, let's see what this is all about.'

"I can't explain what happened to me when I strapped that thing on. I felt like some alien spirit had taken over my body. I was half man, half woman. I thrust my pelvis out and pushed that thing inside him. It was exhilarating. Afterward, however, I felt like I'd had too much chocolate, a little sick.

"He said it hurt. Now we do anal sex only if I say, 'Yeah, honey, really I want it, I'm into it tonight, really.'"

Visual Aids

Erotic DVDs and videos are sex toys, too. They are often used to stimulate arousal during masturbation. And many couples use them as part of foreplay. Erotic films fuel fantasies, improve technique, suggest new ways of having sex—and they can empower women, too.

There is another world of porn—the seriously hard-core stuff that men watch alone, now mostly over the Internet. Women are rarely aroused by this material. Men who spend a lot of time engrossed in it aren't having a lot of partner sex. So it's not an area of importance to us here.

EIGHT PORN FILMS WOMEN LOVE

- *9¹/₂ Weeks*, a mainstream film about S/M.

- *Kama Sutra*, a modern Indian erotic film by director Mira Nair.

- *Last Tango in Paris*, Marlon Brando before he got fat, in the hottest anal-sex film ever.

- *Deep Throat*, the fellatio classic.

- *Emmanuelle*, the ultimate coming-of-age film.

- *Edge Play*, director Veronica Hart's rape fantasy.

- *Three Daughters*, director Candida Royalle's cunnilingus masterpiece.

- *The New Devil in Miss Jones*, starring Jenna Jameson in the best film ever made about a sexually empowered woman.

Tasty stuff

Honey dust, edible body paint, flavored condoms, edible panties—sex has never had so many taste possibilities.

A few caveats before you recklessly toss products into your sex toy shopping cart: Some of these items will be water based, others will be oil based. Oil breaks down latex—so don't use oil-based products with latex condoms. For example, ID Juicy Lubes are all water based and latex safe, but the oils in Wet Fun Flavors Oil Sampler are not latex safe. Read the fine print.

Also, oils—and the bits of paint and flavoring they float—can cling to the inside of your vagina. If you get yeast infections easily, you will probably get one from these products. Many body paints contain oils. The best way to play with them is to paint everything except your vagina—and shower with soap and water before intercourse.

The top-of-the line products are made by Kama Sutra (the company)—and they're beautifully packaged. The ones that are supposed to taste good actually do. Other brands are hit-and-miss. In fact, some "edible body paints" are edible only in the strictest sense: Eating them won't kill you. But you may gag.

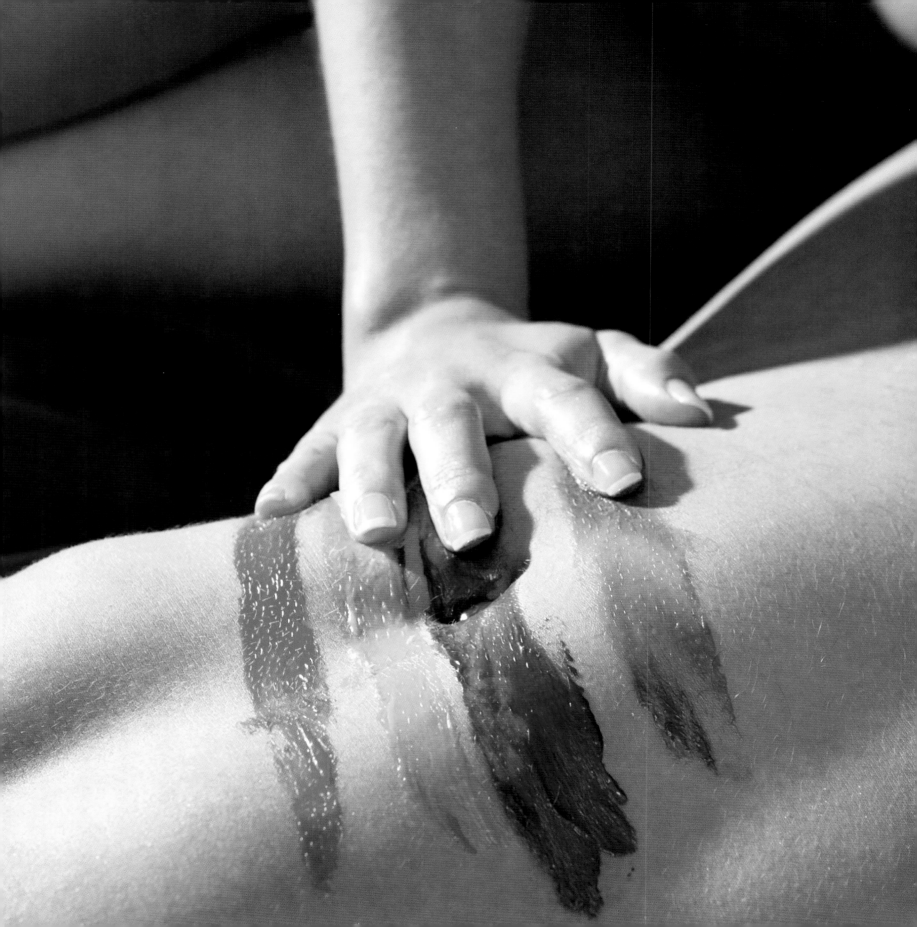

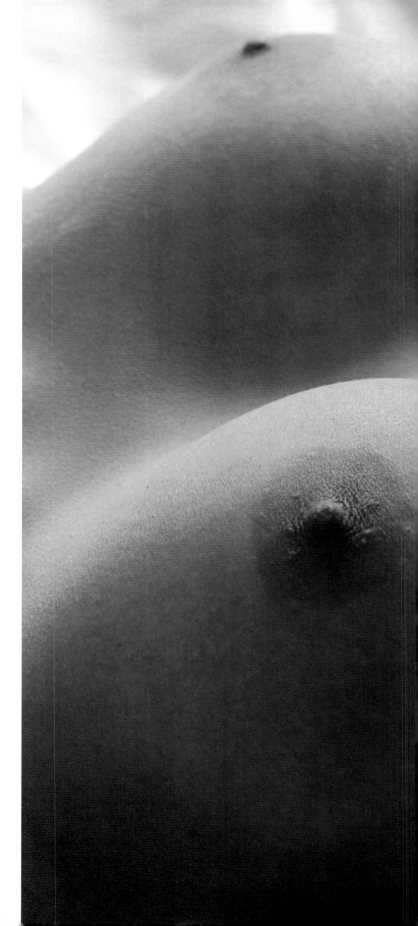

THE INDISPENSABLE SEX GARNISH

Honey Dust, a light, silky, edible dust of honey, has been used in India since ancient times as a natural skin treatment. The dust floats on water. The subtle honeysuckle scent blends with the honey for a delicious aroma. Dip the handmade feather applicator into the dust. Lightly powder your lover's body wherever you plan to lick—and enjoy a delicious sensual sex experience.

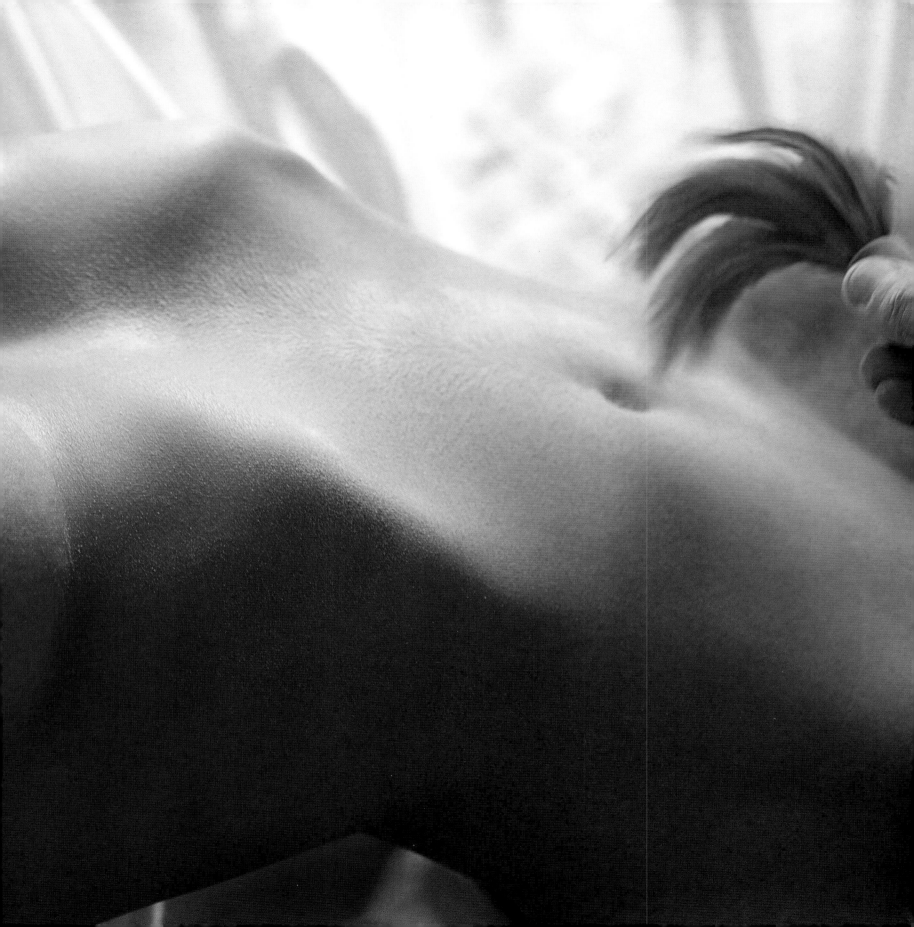

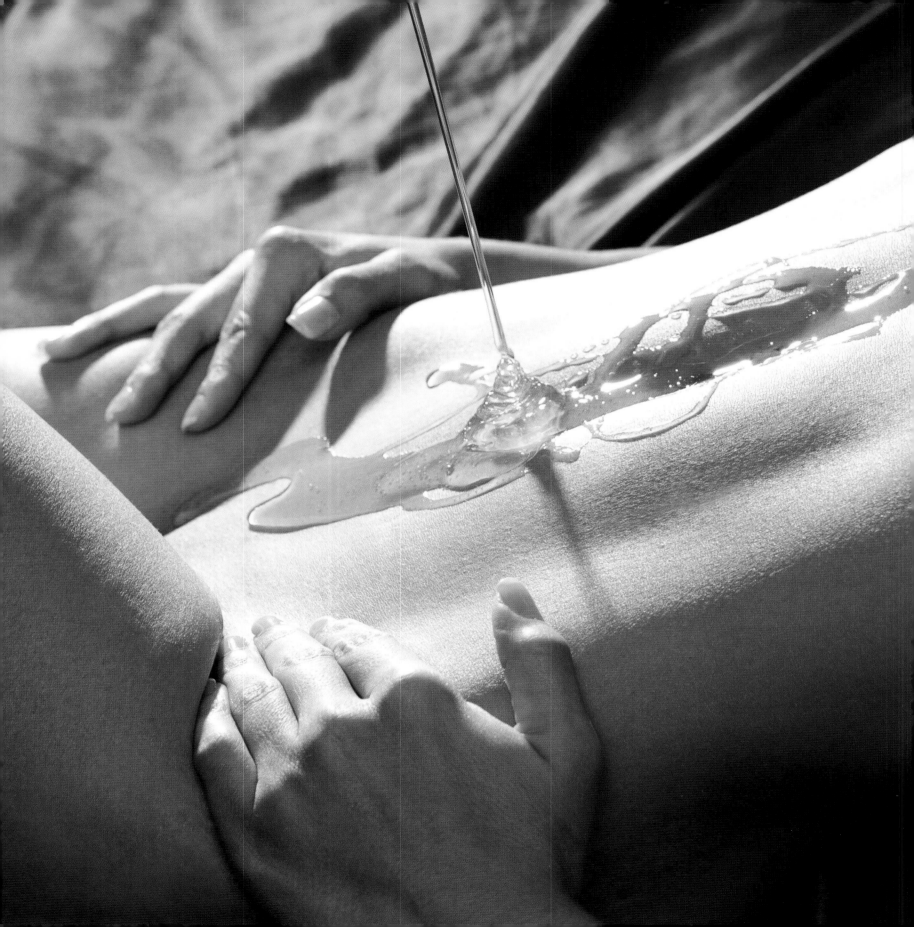

THE RUNNER-UP

Do you think chocolate is as good as (or, the goddess forbid, better than) sex? Try combining the two.

Kama Sutra makes the *Lover's Paintbox*, a set of three smooth, creamy, chocolate body paints, in dark, milk, and white chocolate. The beautiful box resembles an artist's paint box, includes a natural bristle paintbrush and the three flavors in attractive glass jars. The tasty chocolate contains milk and butter and requires refrigeration after opening. It's not sticky—and licks off nicely.

The same company markets edible *Massage Cream* fortified with vitamin E from wheat germ oil. The four delicate flavors are:

Honey Almond, a nice and mild aromatic blend;

Vanilla Crème, sweet and rich;

Cool Mint, refreshing;

and *Raspberry Crème*, really tastes like raspberries.

Anal Toys

Sex toys are a good way to prepare for anal intercourse. Or you can use them for anal masturbation.

Butt plugs, also called anal plugs, are typically diamond-shaped with a thin neck and a flared base, which prevents them from slipping into the rectum. The bulge in the middle stimulates his prostate.

Anal beads cause the sphincter muscles to contract, which can stimulate orgasm in men and women. Beads come in all sizes and materials. They are simply a series of beads knotted into place along a string with a ring on the end.

Anal dildos are a slimmer version of the dildo. They come in several sizes. You can use them to simulate anal intercourse—or, of course, to prepare your body for receiving it.

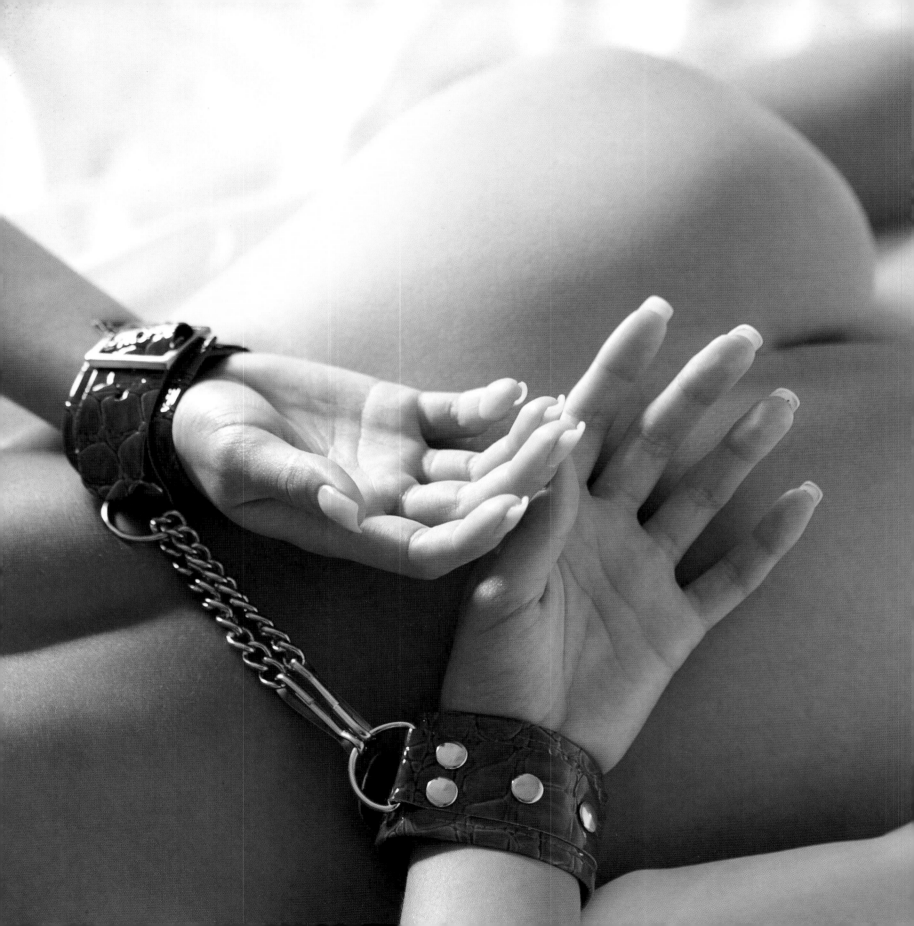

SEX GAMES

Sex in America keeps getting kinkier.

Some sociologists and psychologists believe that kink has always existed and has just come out from behind closed doors. Others say that, yes, of course, kink was always there, but the behaviors are definitely proliferating as ordinary people try what they see in videos, DVDs, and online. They say that "kink" is more commonly practiced in average middle-American bedrooms than ever before. Increasing numbers—between 30 and 60 percent—of "vanilla" couples (those who limit their sex lives to traditional activities) are looking for the hot-fudge sauce, whipped cream, and berries. A decade ago, men were more likely than women to push for a little bondage, a bit of spanking, some S/M games.

Today she may be the one asking: Will you tie me up? Spank me? Whip me with your belt?

The longer a couple have been together, the more likely that one or both will suggest some kinky activity to add spice to their sex lives. Kink seems to be a natural sex-life progression for many couples. If you are ready to give kink a try, agree to play by the "safe, sane, and consensual rules" espoused by the serious lifestylers.

The Rules of the Game

- Agree to the basics, such as, for example, no real pain, or nothing that leaves marks.

- Set a time limit for the amount of time you will "play."

- Designate your roles—and responsibilities.
  Does the master or mistress make the slave come?
  Or forbid that?

- Select a "safe word" that signals "stop." Most couples select something other than "no," because saying "no" while meaning "yes" is part of the fantasy. Choose "peanut butter" or "roses," anything that tells your partner: Okay, it's not play anymore.

S/M or Power Games

S/M, shorthand for sadomasochism, is basically a power exchange between consensual partners. One partner plays the dominant role to the other's submissive. The exchange is acted out through mutually agreed-upon games defined by the power terms listed above.

Not all games will involve the use of belts, paddles, whips. He may, for example, like to be verbally humiliated or forced to kneel before her and beg for release. She may, for example, want to be tied and lightly whipped on her inner thighs and then allowed to masturbate for release.

There are endless scenarios, many incorporating bondage and the use of spanking and whipping instruments and other sex toys.

Why do some people thrill at these games?

Some people enjoy surrendering power now and then, just as others find pleasure in assuming that power. Many couples like to "switch," or take turns playing the dominant and submissive roles. For other people, S/M represents an erotic challenge. They take their own personal erotic experience and the sexual relationship to a new level via these games. And S/M allows some men and women to act out repressed feelings of guilt and shame about their sexuality in a safe and healthy way.

But for many couples, S/M is just a new and different way to play sexually. They like a lot of stimulation and variety in their sex lives. S/M gives them something new without having to switch partners.

How do you know whether or not you would like S/M?

Incorporate a little "rough play" into your lovemaking. Start with love bites, slaps, and pinches. Hold her (or his) nipples between your teeth and bite down gently. Administer little biting kisses to your lover's inner thighs. Slap her (or his) buttocks during intercourse.

If this kind of rough play turns you (and your lover) on, move to the next level. Rent a video or a DVD featuring S/M. Start a dialogue with your lover. Are you on the same page about what is hot and what is definitely not?

If you need more inspiration, go online together. Visit a sex toy store and see how you each respond to the leather and rubber, the nipple clamps and floggers. If you're both still into the game, it's time to draw up your own rules.

Can you play the power game without pain?

Role-playing involves no bondage, discipline, or pain. It's all about acting a part. The couple in a popular yogurt commercial—she's the French maid, he's her wealthy employer—are role-playing. She sits on his lap, spooning yogurt into his mouth, and making suggestive comments. And how interesting that the concept is so mainstream it's used to sell yogurt!

Couples pretending to be strangers meeting in a bar are role-playing, too. And that is a sexy thing to do, because it takes them back to the beginning when they had just met, everything was new, and they had more questions about each other than answers. Role-playing works in two ways: It connects us to who we were when we were new to each other—or it helps us be who we never were.

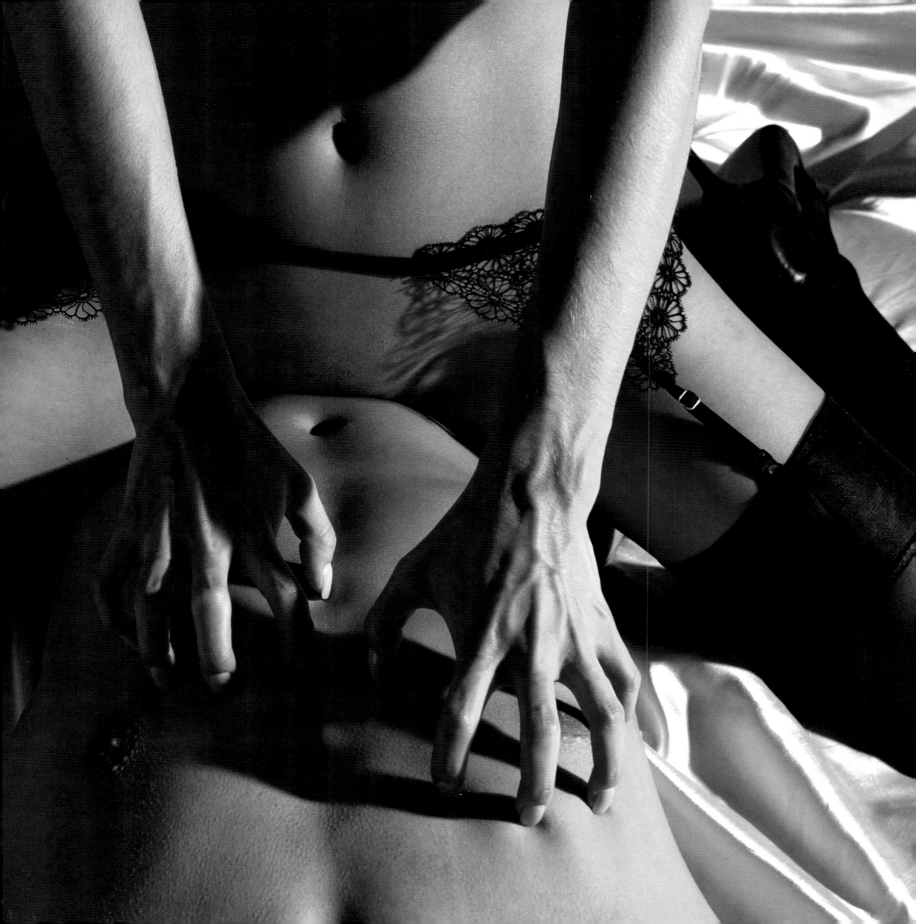

MISTRESS/SLAVE

If you've never played an S/M game before, here are some suggestions to get you started. This is mistress/slave, but you could flip the genders.

Make your slave strip for you while you remain clothed. Order him to touch your genitals without seeing them by insisting that he can only put a hand up your skirt or inside your pants.

Order him to be a voyeur with his hands behind his back while you masturbate as though you were alone.

Make him strip, then blindfold and (Velcro) handcuff him. Tease his penis. Bring him to the point of near orgasm with your hand and/or mouth. Stop. Do it again. Don't bring him to orgasm until he is crazy with desire.

If you're playing that game as master/slave, also tease her to the point of orgasm over and over again. Then masturbate yourself. Ejaculate on her. Untie her and tell her to use your ejaculate as a lubricant and bring herself to orgasm.

Tell her she will be "punished" if she doesn't reach orgasm within a certain time limit, say five minutes.

These are powerful games, not for everyone, but very exciting if they are for you.

TIE AND TEASE

Get into a comfortable position. For most people, that's sitting up in bed with back against the headboard, arms outstretched to the sides, wrists lightly fastened to the headboard.

Use gentle restraints such as Velcro handcuffs or loosely tied silk scarves or ties. Don't use metal handcuffs or tight knots. The bound person should be able to work his or her hands free. It's a game, not an arrest.

Tease your partner with light kisses and touches. Use oils and lotions. Run a feather lightly up and down his or her inner thighs. Fondle nipples through a silk scarf. Put rose petals on your finger pads and massage your lover's nipples and genitals. Be creative in your use of sensual materials.

Vary the pattern of teasing strokes, from passionate kisses now to gentle caresses later.

Focus on the pleasure points: nipples, on both men and women, inner thighs, backs of knees, ears, neck, the line from the navel down to the pubis, and the genitals, including the perineum.

Bring your partner to the brink of orgasm, pull back, tease again.

Unleash the orgasm(s) — manually, orally, and/or via intercourse.

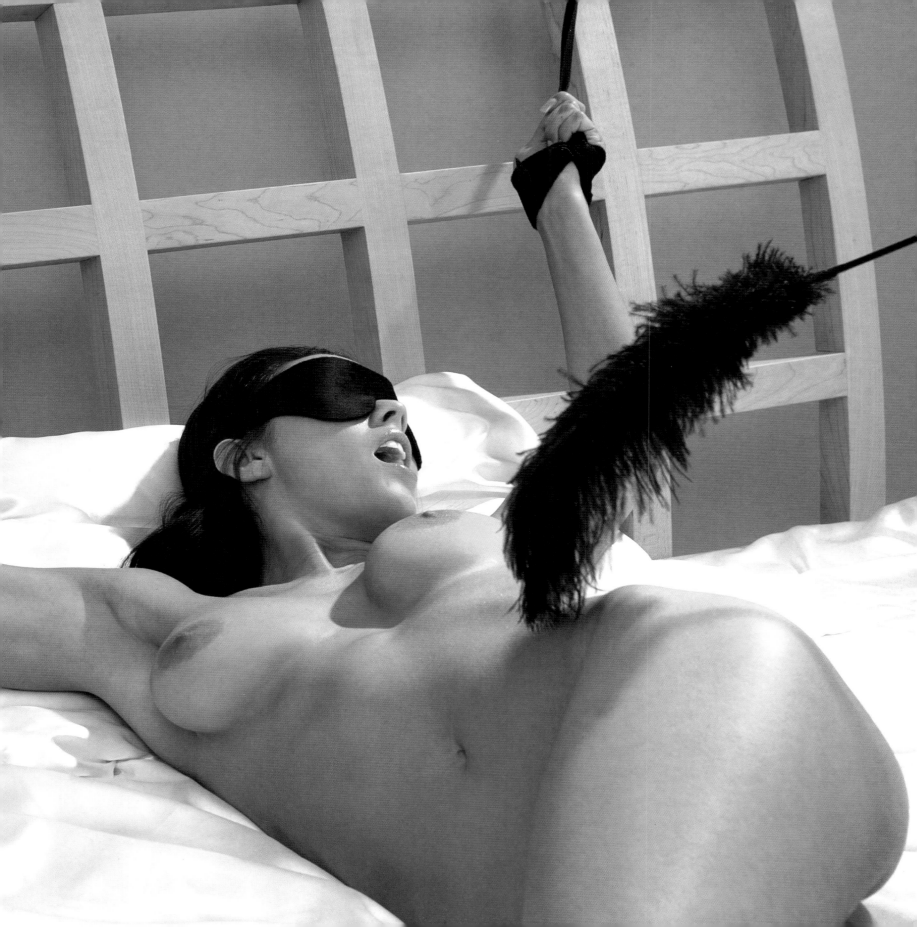

Erotic Spanking

Judging by the numerous Web sites, magazines, videos, and DVDs—and the support groups dedicated to practitioners—erotic spanking is a very popular sex game. And "erotic spanking" is exactly what it sounds like it is: spanking for the sexual gratification of either or both lovers. Some people regard spanking as one of several S/M games to play, while serious devotees don't play any other games. They only spank.

Almost everyone has received or administered—or both—a few swats to the buttocks during lovemaking, typically intercourse.

You can spank with your hand or use an implement such as a ruler, hairbrush, paddle, belt, kitchen spatula—or, for the serious spanker and spankee, a cane or a crop. Sometimes the blows are delivered to the bare buttocks, sometimes the spankee wears panties or his bikini briefs. Positions for spanking include:

- over the knees or across the lap;

- lying facedown on a bed;

- stooped over the back of a chair;

- bending forward, hands on knees;

- kneeling on a bed or an ottoman, stooped over with hands on the floor;

- on all fours.

Many couples combine spanking with role-playing. The naughty schoolgirl (or boy), the daddy (or mommy), teacher and pupil are favorite roles. In these role-playing games, couples may use spanking as a form of "punishment." Costumes are often part of the play. The schoolgirl may wear kneesocks and a miniskirt; the maid, stocking, garter belt, and a sheer apron.

Erotic spanking requires skill—and a measured hand. Deliver a blow deemed "too hard" and you kill the mood. Before you even start to spank, lay your partner across your lap, lift her skirt or slide your hand inside his briefs and gently caress the quivering flesh.

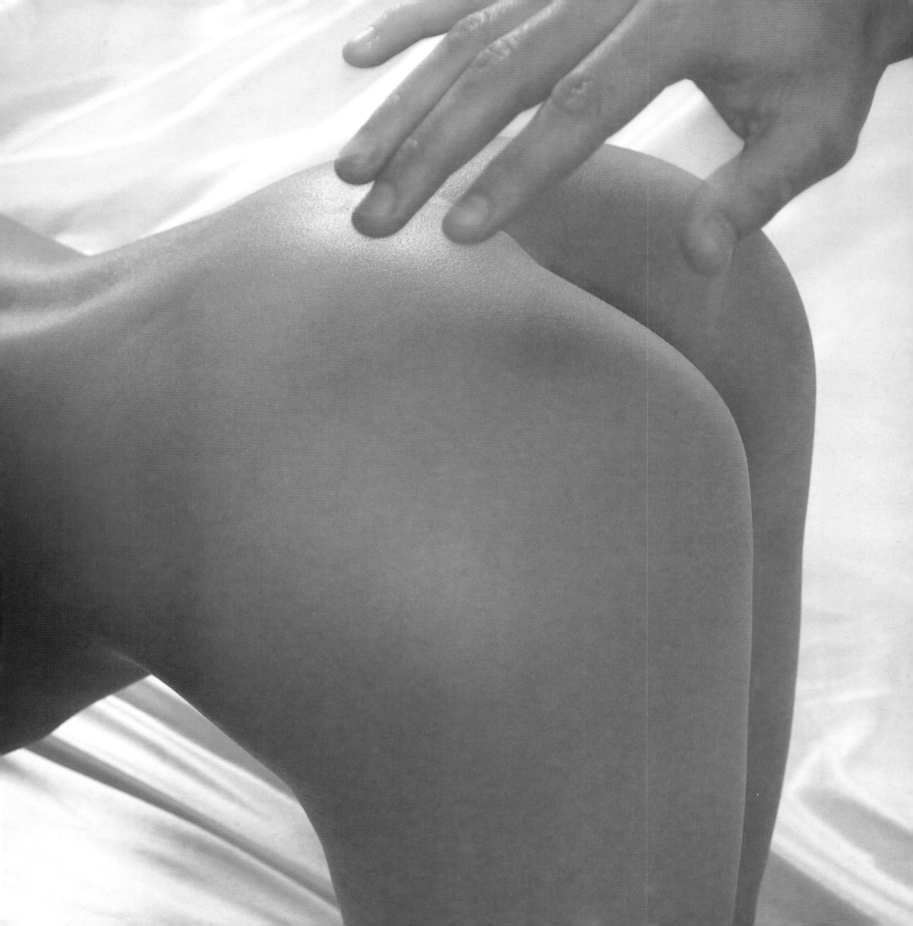

SPANKING VARIATIONS

Spread your lover's bottom cheeks with one hand and softly spank the anal area with two or three fingers of the other hand.

Relax your wrist so that your hand works like a paddle.

Spread your fingers when you smack rather than holding them together as you probably have been doing.

These moves create different sensations for the willing recipient.

FANTASY

Fantasy is a nearly universal experience, a mental aphrodisiac with amazing powers. Sometimes it is a conscious process, sometimes not. But if you are not satisfied with your sex life and you aren't using fantasy to create and sustain arousal, you are missing something: the fastest and easiest route to arousal or orgasm.

Shame or fear of being "abnormal" keeps some people from acknowledging, sharing, or enjoying their fantasies. Fantasizing a sexual act—such as a homosexual encounter, violent sex, or group sex—doesn't mean that you want to do it. Many people, for example, fantasize homosexual encounters without wanting to have sex with someone of the same gender in real life. Unless you have nothing but violent fantasies and can't be aroused any other way, your fantasies are normal, whatever that means.

Use them, enjoy them, don't take them too seriously.

Recent studies indicate that men and women now have fantasies that are more alike than they were twenty years ago. According to Nancy Friday, author of *Women on Top* and other books about sexual fantasies, women's fantasies have become more graphic and overtly sexual and aggressive. Don't be afraid or ashamed of these fantasies.

SPANKING

Warm up your lover's bottom with light slaps until her cheeks flush. Stop. Caress his buttocks. Repeat the slaps with a slightly firmer touch. Stop. Caress and massage the warm flesh.

Whether using your hand or an implement, maintain a steady but not too intense pace. Never exert too much force. You have to be more careful with an implement, because you can't feel the pressure being exerted in your own hand. Remember, the quantity of slaps, not the force, creates the erotic excitement.

Where you direct those light blows makes a difference, too. The lower buttocks, along the crease where they meet your lover's legs, and the full sides of his bottom are very sensitive. Don't strike the tailbone!

What is the number-one question

about sexual fantasies?

"Are my fantasies 'normal'?"

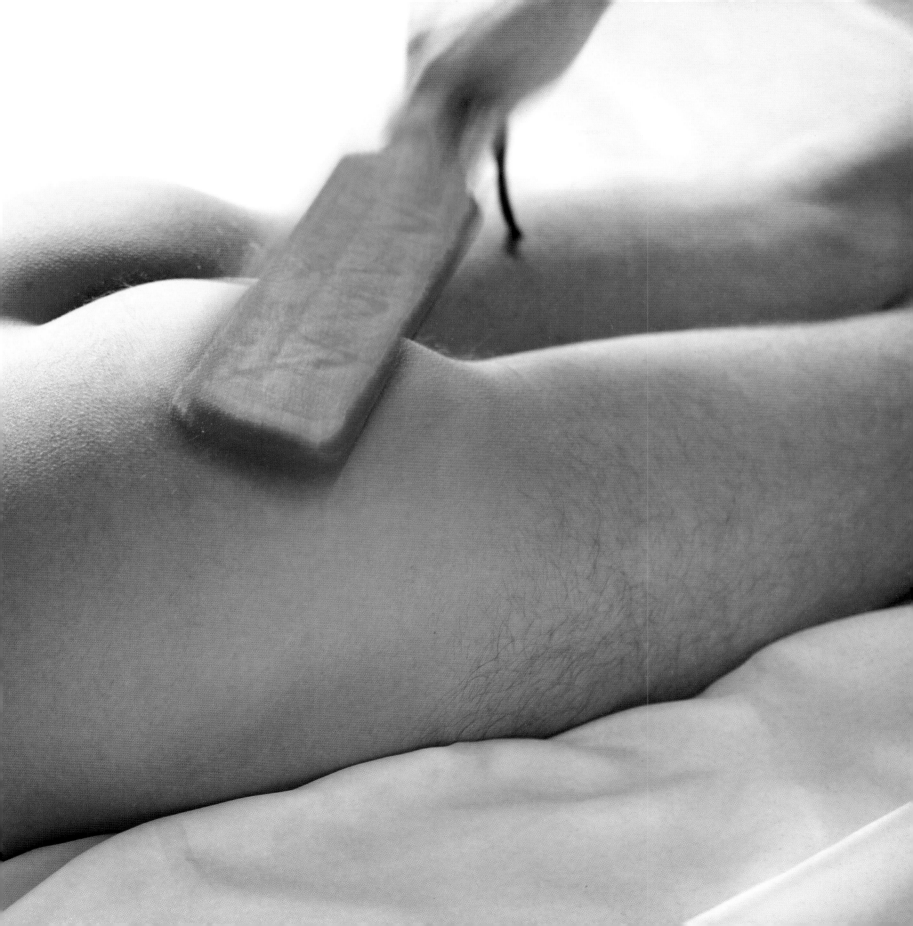

A COUPLE'S STORY

In her dreams, Megan lubricated at the sound of the leather belt's being pulled through its loops. Tremors ran through her body as he tested the belt against his hand. Thwack! She is tied to the bed, spread-eagle. The first strokes are soft, almost caressing whacks of the belt, because he knows how to make her crave the pain. The sound changes as the strokes grow harder. Her body is covered in slick sweat now. And the belt hits with a wet thud . . .

The dream always ended the same way, in orgasm. She woke with her hand inside her, panting and sweating, the stings she had dreamed disappearing as the contractions of her orgasm ebbed away.

Beside her Brian snored, sleeping soundly, unaware.

Sometimes she taunted him, but he didn't seem to get her point. *Spank me! You don't like what I said? Make me take it back!* He laughed. Or she picked up his pants, discarded on the bedroom floor, slowly removed the belt from its loops, and lightly struck the palm of her hand with it. Once. Twice. He looked up, frowned quizzically at her and said, "Okay, I should pick up my own clothes."

They'd been together seven years. She had the itch to have her ass smacked by a belt. And she couldn't tell him that. She'd been craving that smack for as long as she could remember. The dream about the belt had been recurring since she was a teenager. But why? Her parents hadn't even spanked her with an open hand, much less a belt. And she couldn't tell him any of that.

She wanted the belt, she didn't know why—and she certainly didn't know how to ask for it.

One night she woke before the orgasm started. Hot, wet, unbearably in need, she rolled over and climbed on top of Brian. He came to life—and moaned, barely opening his eyes, as he thrust energetically up to meet her. She rode him to a furious climax, the belt hitting her rhythmically in her mind.

"What was that all about?" he asked her in the morning.

"I had a dream," she said, without looking into his eyes.

Several days later, they were sitting on the floor in front of a splendid fire, wineglasses in hand, and he asked, "The dream? Another man?"

Her face felt hot, maybe from the fire. Stricken, she looked hard into her husband's eyes. He was hurt, confused. She had to say something.

"It was a belt," she said. "Your belt."

"A belt?"

And she watched him figure it out slowly, the thought process excruciating. She could see him remembering. *Spank me.* He was getting it.

"A belt," he said.

She was hot with shame, with desire.

"A belt," he said again, his voice stronger, more confident.

He pulled her into his arms, kissed her roughly, whispered in her ear, "You want the belt."

She trembled in response.

"Take off your pants," he said.

Lying over the pillows, her ass quivering in the air, she finally received the belt she had been dreaming about.

THE TOP TEN FANTASY SCENARIOS

Many people have a "favorite friend" fantasy, that erotic scenario guaranteed to arouse during masturbation or when arousal subsides during lovemaking. The friend will likely be in one of the following categories:

1. Making love with someone other than your regular partner—the most common fantasy for both men and women. (Yes, women, too, fantasize during lovemaking.)

2. The forbidden partner—someone of a different race or class, a relative, a friend's spouse, your boss or personal assistant.

3. Multiple partners, typically sex with your lover and another person. (For men, the "two women" fantasy is a favorite.)

4. The romantic fantasy—sex with your partner in an idyllic place such as the beach at sunset.

5. Spontaneous stranger encounter—such as the "zipless fuck" popularized by author Erica Jong in the classic novel *Fear of Flying*, in which strangers meet on a train, for example, and fall upon each other, their clothes falling magically away.

6. Forced sex—sometimes called "the rape fantasy," and actually common to both men and women. (The fantasy signifies a desire to have sex without guilt and responsibility, not actually a desire to be raped.)

7. "Taboo" sex acts such as having sex in a public place or practicing S/M.

8. Exhibitionist or voyeuristic fantasies in which one is having sex while being watched or watching someone else have sex. (A common version of this fantasy for men is watching a wife or a girlfriend have sex with someone else.)

9. Homosexual encounter.

10. Sex with a celebrity.

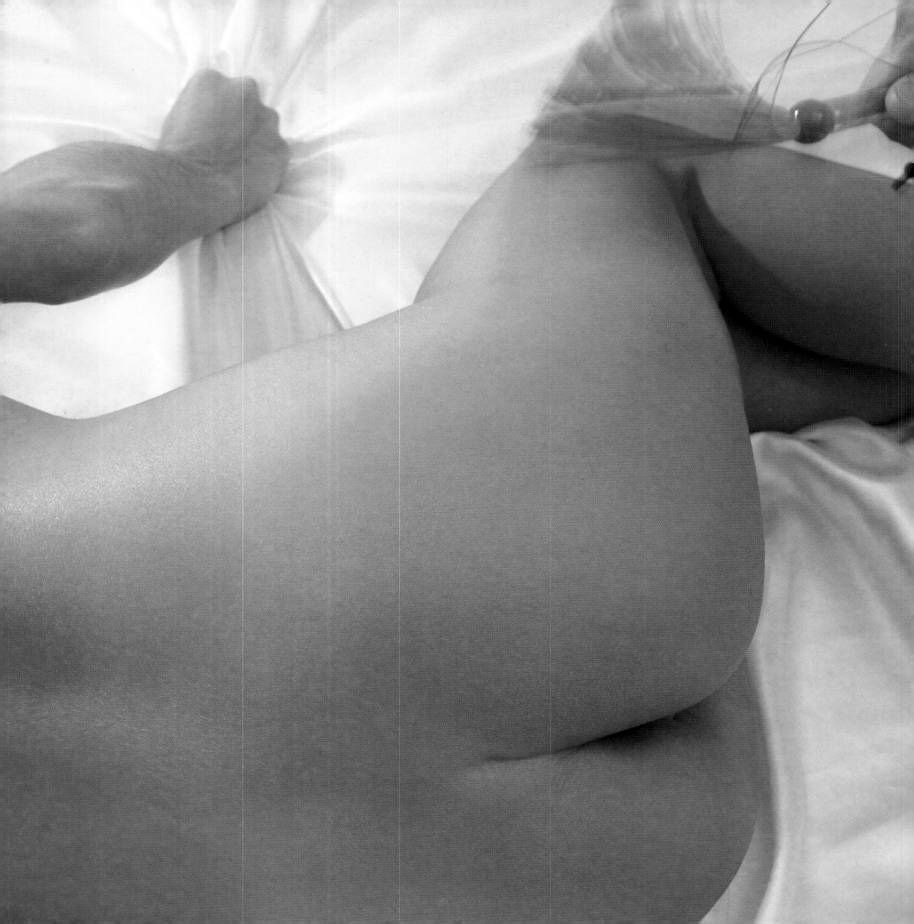

FANTASY AS MENTAL FOREPLAY

Keep a fantasy notebook and jot down erotic ideas or scenarios that excite you. Don't censor yourself. It's okay to fantasize anything.

Once you have developed a story line—something as basic as sex on a tropical island or as complex as an S/M scene set in a dungeon—use that fantasy as mental foreplay. Before having sex with your partner, pull out the fantasy.

And together develop some fantasies based on memories of your shared erotic past.

Go back to the first time you made love or a particularly thrilling encounter. Now use those fantasies regularly as mental foreplay.

Making it happen

You want to act out a fantasy with your lover?

Start with something easy, such as, phone sex.

Ask the classic question "What are you wearing?" Get a very detailed answer.

"I'm wearing a black-silk shirt, unbuttoned so that the tops of my breasts show. The fabric clings to me. My skirt is tight and white. I'm not wearing any underwear. My shoes are three-inch black stilettos. My legs are bare and shiny. I oiled them."

Now suggest a sex act you'd like to perform on your lover dressed this way.

"I want to kneel in front of you, push up your skirt, and go down on you."

After that, suggest role-playing. Play gigolo/rich lady or call girl/businessman. Dress your parts. Meet as strangers in a bar and negotiate the deal. Exchange money. State the sexual terms. Stay in character as you go home to act it out.

Or take turns playing each other's favorite film characters. Remember how Ross in the hit show *Friends* tapped into the collective fantasy consciousness of a generation when he asked Rachel to dress as Princess Leia from the first *Star Wars* series? Even meeting him in bed wearing a feathered mask and high heels can make you feel new to each other.

Acting out fantasies (that are mutually acceptable and arousing) is a great way to shake things up sexually. When you act out a part, you let go of attitudes and inhibitions that were holding you back. You may be surprised how much you like—and are freed by—sexual theater when you try it.

What if your partner says, "No"?

Negotiate with your reluctant lover.

Ask: What can we do to make this fantasy acceptable to you and still hot to me?

Try to develop a fantasy scenario together that has the elements you find arousing without making your lover feel silly or turned off. Write the script together. Give your lover the greater more input.

Even the most reluctant fantasy player usually gets aroused if the script is right.

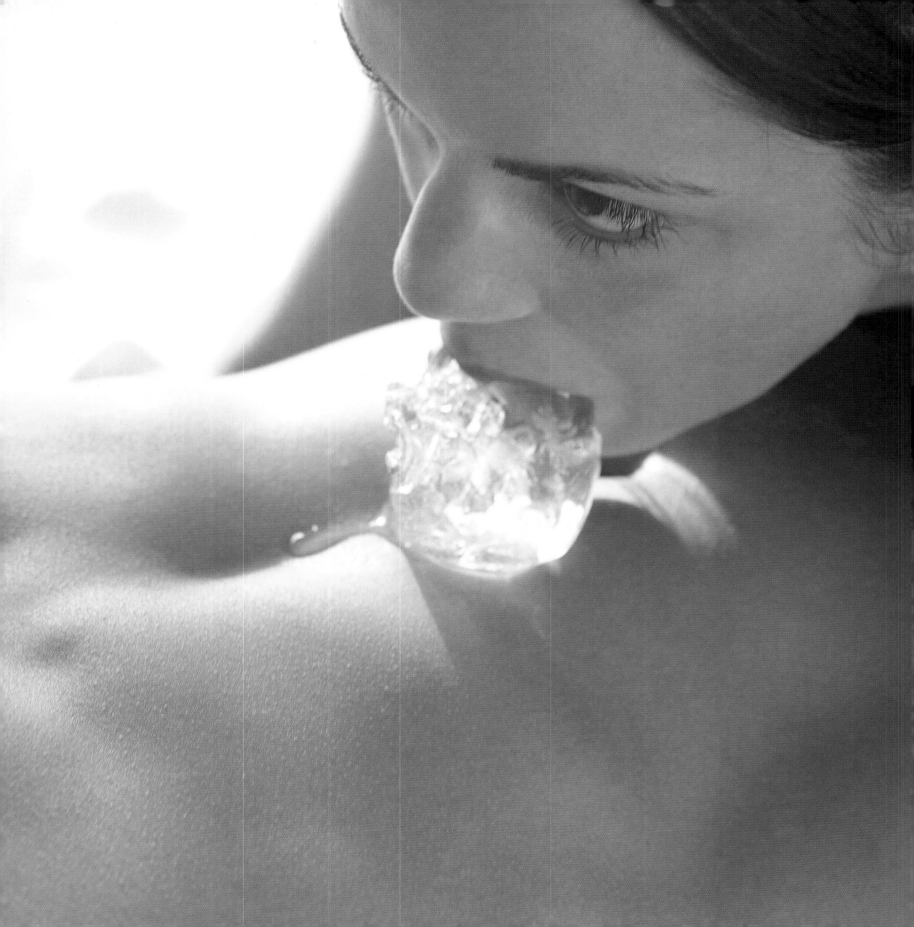

THE FIVE FANTASY RULES

A few simple rules will keep you out of trouble with your lover.

1. Never admit to fantasizing about your partner's siblings, parents, best friends. If you've already done that and your lover is mad, your story is: "I was just trying to get a reaction out of you." Stick to that story.

2. Don't admit that you fantasize about someone else while the two of you make love—unless you know that your partner is aroused by fantasies of you with someone else. Otherwise this is the you're-really-in-trouble-now fantasy. In truth, everyone fantasizes about another partner occasionally—but only fools acknowledge that.

3. Don't share a fantasy about a man with a big penis if your man has a small one—and is self-conscious about his size. The same holds true for women's breasts. Take your partner's best features and weave them into a fantasy you share.

4. Fantasizing together out loud during sex can be very hot. But make your lover the object of your fantasy.

5. Don't ridicule a fantasy that your lover shares with you. Imagine you are the only one who admits after years of secret fantasizing that you want to have sex on the steps of the Lincoln Memorial—only to have your significant other laugh.

Technique Tip

THE NEGOTIATED FANTASY

Break the questionable fantasy down into content elements. If your lover, for example, fantasizes a bondage scenario and you object to that, ask yourself why. Are you upset because the sexual imagery is politically incorrect? Talk through those issues and try to get them out of your sex life. It helps if you understand that bondage—again, for example—represents freedom from responsibility.

Use costumes and props. If you love the television show *Desperate Housewives*, dress as sexy Gabrielle and have him play the young, shirtless, and sweaty gardener she seduces. Costumes really are important. It's hard to pretend you're a glamorous movie star or a cruel domme if you don't even put on lipstick and heels.

Look for ways to compromise and camouflage. You fantasize being dominated. Call it "swept off your feet," conjuring that famous image of Rhett carrying Scarlett up the staircase.

Work from a real script. That adds to the sense of play and makes the whole process seem less embarrassing somehow. If you're having trouble getting in touch with your inner erotic creativity, borrow from a novel or a film.

Exhibitionism/Voyeurism

Voyeurs like to watch and exhibitionists like to be watched. There is a little of each in most of us. Women who flaunt their cleavage or legs are exhibitionists. Couples who make out in bars are exhibitionists—and the people watching every kiss and touch are voyeurs. Everyone who has lived in a high-rise apartment has looked in someone else's windows. And did you ever notice how many of those people don't have drapes or blinds?

Why do these behaviors appeal to so many of us?

Showing or doing something a little private (and thus naughty) in a public space is exhilarating. So is sneaking a peek at something you weren't meant—or don't feel entitled—to see. Obviously, "flashers," men who expose their penises in public, have taken the concept too far. They are creepy, not titillating.

Technique Tip

SHOWING IT OFF

Stop avoiding PDAs (public displays of affection). In fact, turn up the heat on them.

Touch each other in barely legal places—for example, run your finger inside her blouse and under the edge of her bra or rest your hand briefly on his trouser-covered penis. Dark and luxurious bars are perfect places for these games. Get a table or a booth out of traffic or snag the end barstools, preferably with one against a wall—and certainly game-play only during hours when the neighborhood parents are not having burgers with the kids.

Dress sexy. Show some cleavage or an expanse of thigh, legs bare or in black thigh-high stockings with lace tops. (Men, loosen the tie.) Be meticulous about grooming. Couples who have been together awhile fall into lazy habits. Get out of that rut.

I promise you: Cleavage, smooth bare legs, high heels, and a stash of silky thigh-high stockings will improve your sex life.

" Real talk "

"My neighborhood bar is a classy establishment that has been in business for twenty-five years," Susannah says. "Occasionally and late at night some couple uses the last stall in the ladies' room for oral sex. Every now and then you see a man and a woman locked in embrace in the hallway leading to the kitchen. It's that kind of place.

"One night I was sitting on a barstool in the window, waiting for my boyfriend of three years. When he came in, he said I looked beautiful. And he started flirting with me as if we had only just met. I was wearing a soft black-cashmere sweater, green skirt, no stockings, high heels.

"'Do your panties match the top of your skirt?' he asked.

"'You'll just have to find out,' I answered, playing coy.

"He got off his stool, knelt on the floor in front of me, gently opened my knees, peered up my legs to determine the panties were green, then kissed each knee before standing up again.

"We had the hottest sex that night."

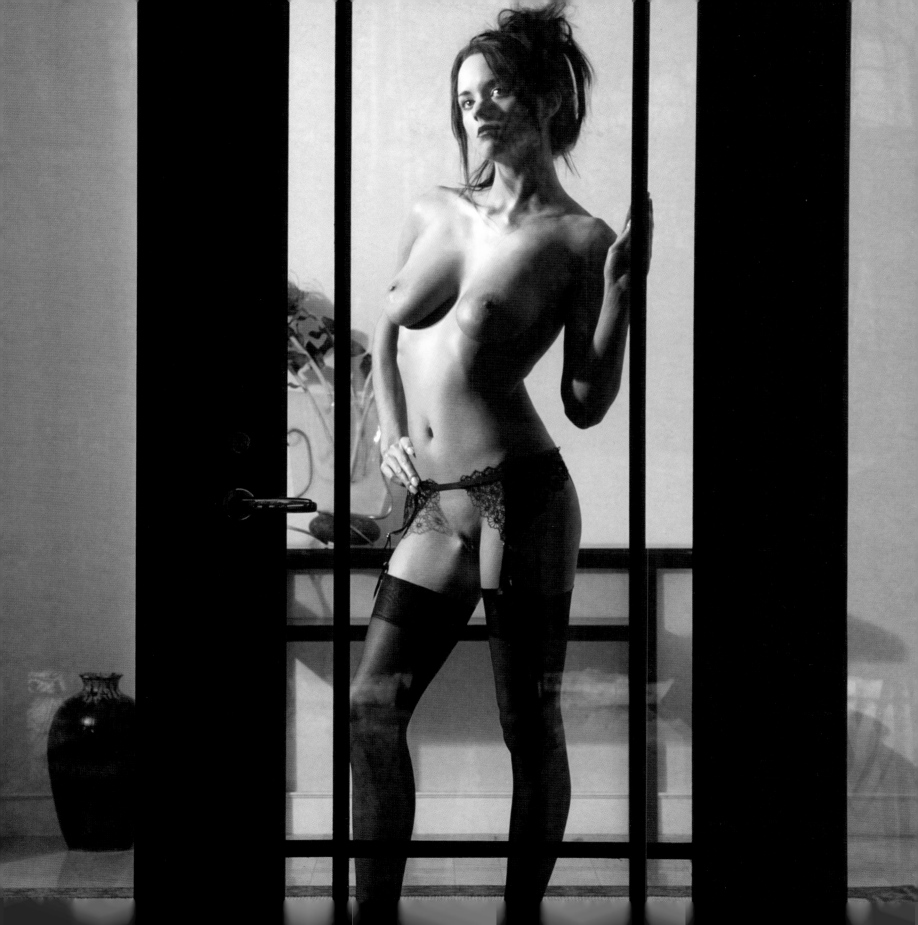

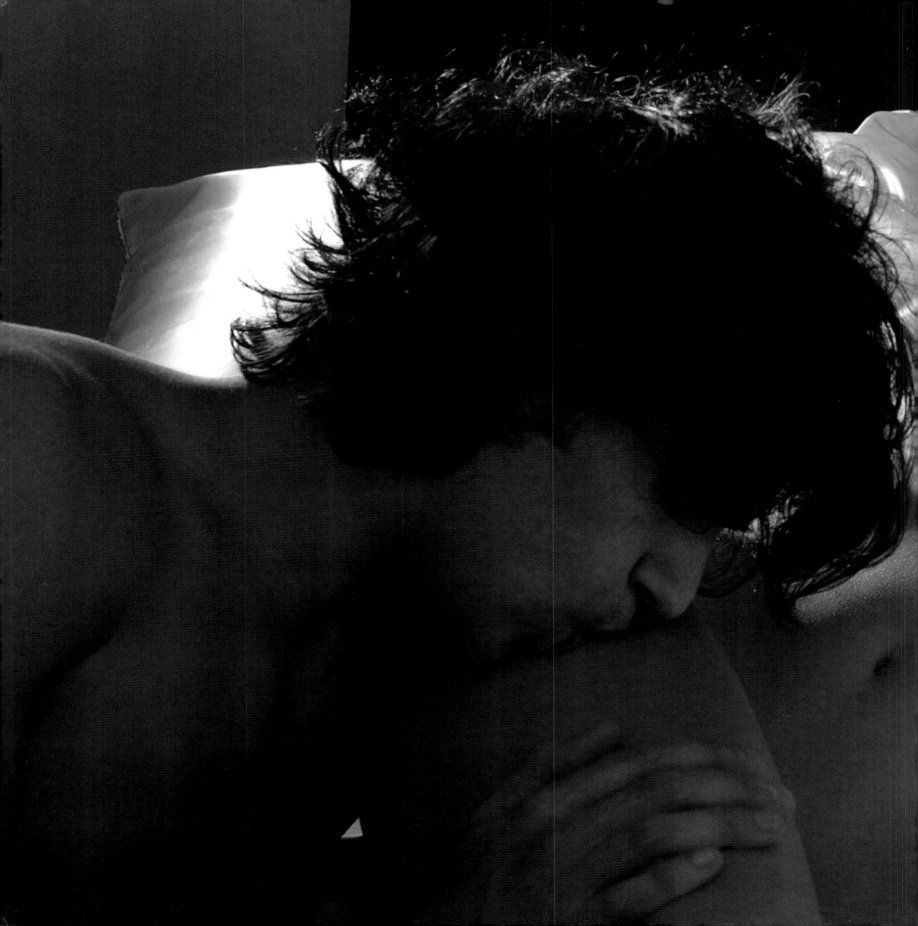

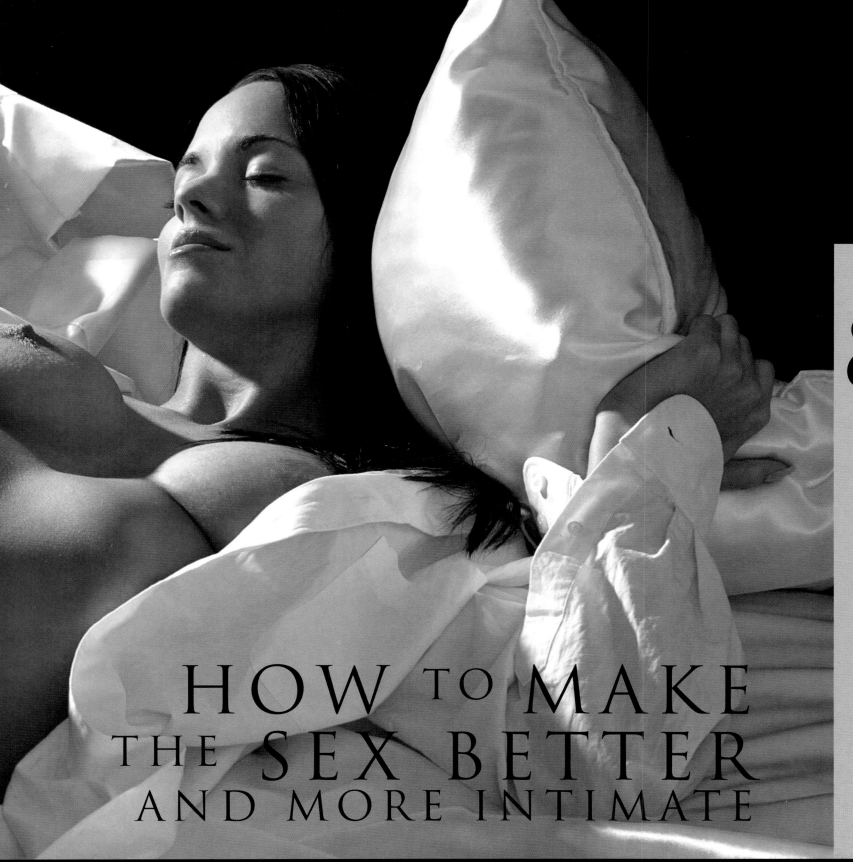

8

HOW TO MAKE
THE SEX BETTER
AND MORE INTIMATE

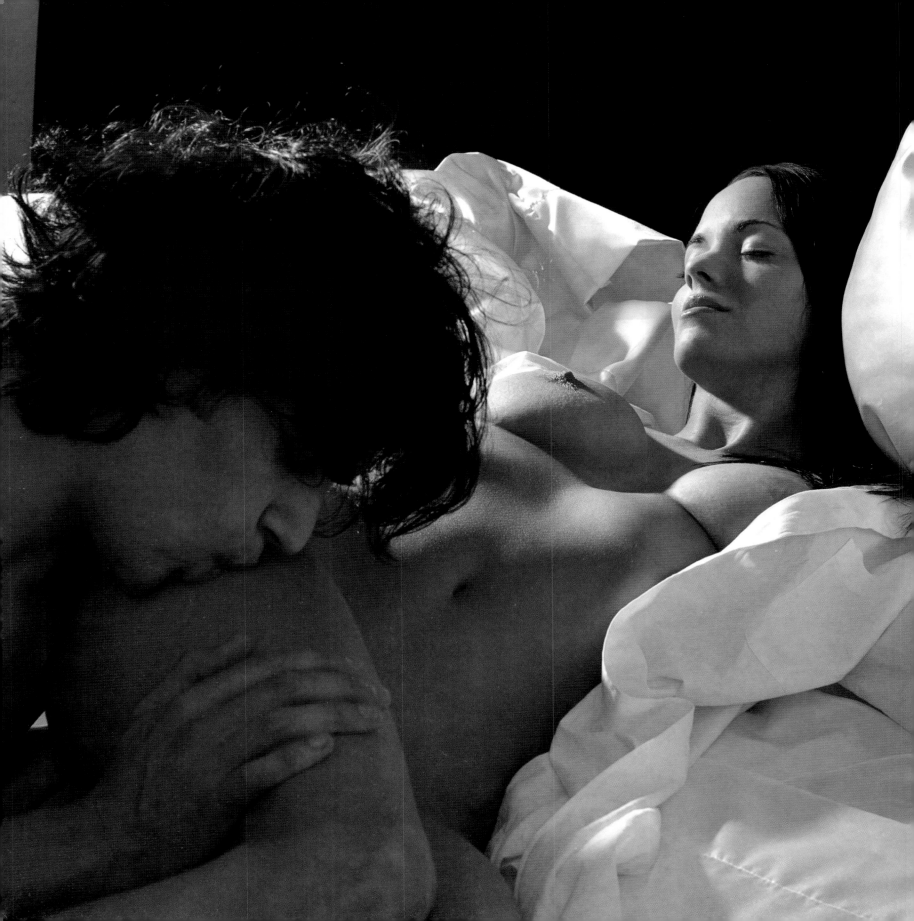

THE LITTLE FIXES

———

"Sex is such an urgent message from our body that sometimes

we call it our soul. Lust carries risks, sexual intimacy has consequences:

It is nature, not a gadget with a warranty.

Nobody would go through it if the rewards were not so magnificent."

— Susie Bright
Author of *Susie Bright's*
Sexual State of the Union

THIS IS NOT a chapter filled with the standard advice for a usual suspects list of sex/relationship ills. If you've come this far into *The Sex Bible*, you love sex, you are an adventurous lover, and you value the intimate connection. You (and your partner) aren't candidates for a Dr. Phil intervention. Every now and then, however, you will need a technique for taking the two of you over a bumpy patch—when libido flags, an erection wilts, an injury or pregnancy must be accommodated.

Or one day you may feel that the sizzle and excitement has temporarily gone from your sex life. Or you may wake up and realize that you have been too stressed, too tired, too busy for sex for too long now. You're missing the passion and excitement of good sex. And you're missing something equally important: the intense intimate connection with your lover that you feel during and after lovemaking.

You want to fix the sex because you miss the pleasure—and crave the intimacy.

Here are the "little fixes" that will put you back on track.

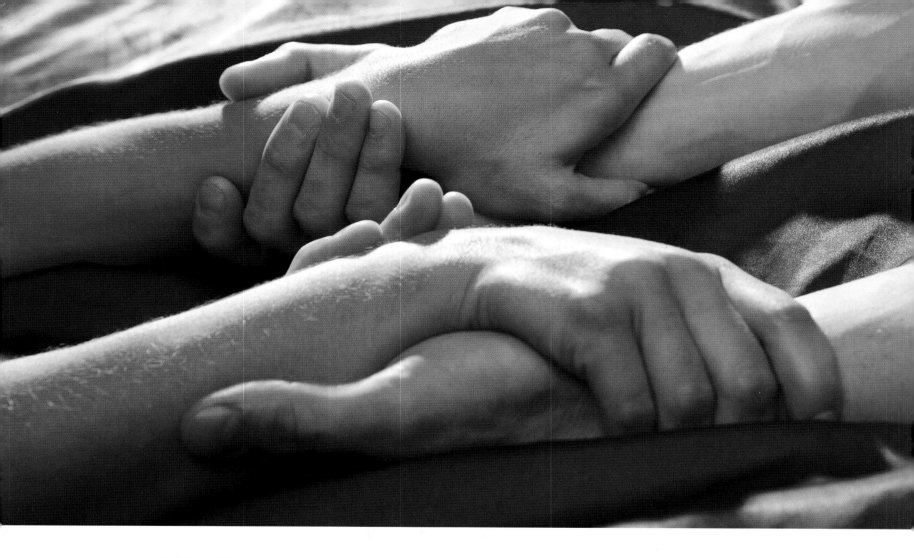

A Familiar Story

Every couple occasionally walks through the valley of sexual boredom. They know each other so well that there seems to be no surprise or mystery left. They press each other's hot spots as surely as if they were entering PIN codes into an ATM. And predictable good sex leading to orgasm is often a very good thing—like getting the cash from that ATM. Sometimes it is exactly what we want from sex.

And sometimes it isn't.

Small changes can make a big difference. If you usually get undressed together, chatting about the events of the day, before falling into bed for sex, try grabbing your lover and groping her (him) through clothes. No talk, just hot kisses.

Change just one aspect of how you "do it"— and you're not predictable anymore.

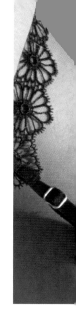

THE TOP FIVE INTIMACY—CREATING SEX TECHNIQUES

These are the best sex techniques for bringing you both emotionally and physically close.

1. *Eyes open kissing.* Keep your eyes open as you kiss, beginning with gentle nibbles and sucks to his lips, one at a time. With the tip of your tongue, flirt with his lips and the tip of his tongue. Then kiss him deeply. (See page 42).

2. *Body stroking.* Use your hands all over, not just on genitals. Alternate long, slow sensuous strokes using the palms of your hands on his chest, back, shoulders, thighs—with playful touches, such as "walking" around his body with the pads of your fingertips. (See page 55.)

3. *Expert fellatio.* Pay loving attention to his penis. Use a variety of techniques—flicking, licking, and swirling your tongue around the head. And don't forget the shaft. (See page 73.)

4. *Hand over heart.* This is simple and incredibly intimate. Put your hand over his heart as he's reaching orgasm. Or place his hand over your heart as you come.

5. *Whispered words.* After orgasm, whisper directly into his ear. Tell him how wonderful he's made you feel and how much you love him. Keep it short and make it real.

Revitalize Your Signature Sex Move

We all have a signature sex move. Maybe it's his kiss on her throat as he caresses her face, or the way she takes his penis in both hands and twists him to ecstasy, or the way she works that Corkscrew Twist during intercourse, or how he holds her hips and locks her gaze as he thrusts deeply. You've got The Move, maybe more than one. It works, but it's predictable.

Shake it up—with the following techniques. And let them inspire you to come up with others, targeted at your signature sex move.

Technique Tip

THE "COME TO PAPA" KISS

If she hasn't been enthusiastic about sex lately, pull back from the deep French kiss, the one that signals your desire for intercourse. Use the tip of your tongue in circles just inside her lips. Tease those lips again and again with the circling tip of your tongue—the way you tease her clitoris. Stop. Suck her lips gently, one at a time. Walk away.

Let her come to you for that French kiss. Now she wants it—and more.

Technique Tip

FLIP YOUR FLICK

While performing fellatio, flick your tongue in places you normally don't. If he expects you to flick rapidly back and forth across the corona, don't go there. Flick the frenulum, the top of the head of the penis, his perineum.

Instead of sucking the head of his penis, suck his testicles.

Move your mouth and tongue in your signature way—but not in the usual places.

Technique Tip

DRESS YOUR TONGUE

Perform cunnilingus while she's wearing a pair of wispy panties. Lick through and around them, but don't put your tongue on her clitoris.

Put rose petals on your finger pads and as you are licking her panties, use your rose-covered fingers to press her inner thighs and labia.

Bring her to orgasm by using the bridge of your nose to massage her clitoris and the surrounding tissue.

Technique Tip

CHANGE YOUR POSITIONS

If the female superior position is your move, vary it by "riding the bull," with one hand in the air, one hand on your clitoris, and an exaggerated riding style. Or lean forward and rub your breasts against his chest, nipple to nipple. Or turn and face his feet.

Change the way you use your favorite orgasm position— and you change the experience for both of you.

If the missionary position is your move, vary it by bringing her knees to her chest and lifting up her buttocks with your hands. You will enter her at a thirty-degree angle— changing the way intercourse feels for both of you.

The two basic "Fix it!" scenarios

When a couple says, "The sex isn't working," they usually mean one of two things:

- She loses her arousal during lovemaking and therefore doesn't reach orgasm.
- He loses his erection during lovemaking.

These two issues do need to be addressed. They aren't hard to fix. And if you don't, one or both of you may start finding excuses for not having sex. The intimate connection will fray. And nobody wants that.

HER AROUSAL/ORGASM

The Orgasm Loop ensures her arousal and orgasm. (See page 149.)

Why is orgasm such a big deal?

For a man—and if we're being honest, for a woman, too—orgasm opens into intimacy.

Orgasm is the most intense personal experience we ever have. Nothing else provides so much pleasure, releases so much tension, leaves us with such a strong sense of well-being—and has the power to enhance our intimate relationships at the same time. The sexual energy that drives orgasm is a great force of nature. The ancient Hindus were wise to worship sexual energy.

Given the power and glory that is orgasm, we shouldn't accept the theory that his orgasm is inevitable while hers is problematic. Why should female orgasm be problematic when women are the possessors of the clitoris, richer with more concentrated nerve endings than any part of his body? Exactly. It shouldn't be a problem at all.

If you use the Orgasm Loop, it won't be.

Once you're back on track, celebrate your new found intimacy.

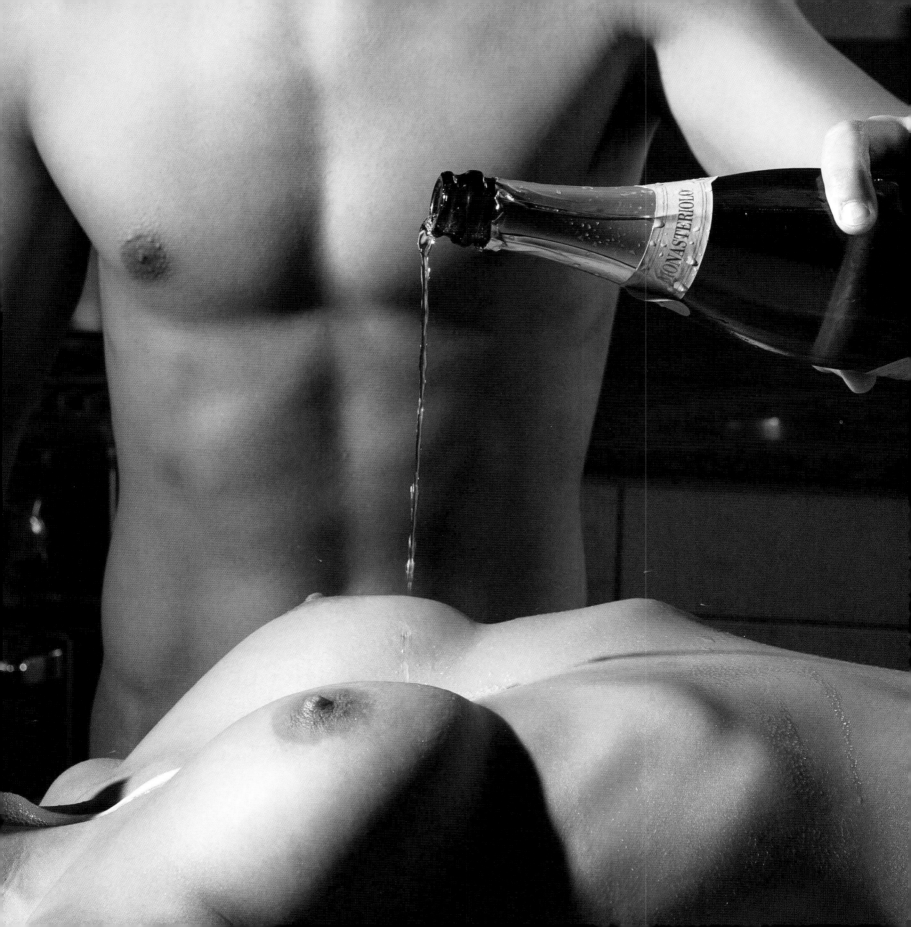

HIS ERECTION LOSS

Fellatio as you typically perform it may not be enough. But this move is almost guaranteed to make him erect—even if he thinks he's lost the will to come back to life. If he's drunk, however, there's probably nothing you can do to counteract the drinks hanging on the end of his penis.

Don't take the blame for that.

Technique Tip

THE PERFECT STAND-UP KISS

The secret to this move: *Combine mouth and firm hand action.*

Hold his penis firmly in one hand. Take it into your mouth, moving the top third of the shaft in and out. Use the fingers of your other hand to stroke his perineum in a light, tickling come-hither fashion.

When he becomes erect, use one hand to do the circular twisting motion described on page 73 at the same time you swirl your tongue around the corona . Pay particular attention to the frenulum . Alternate the swirl with the Butterfly Flick—flicking your tongue back and forth across the corona.

Continue the hand move while taking his testicles into your mouth, one at a time, and sucking lightly. Flick your tongue lightly across his perineum. Go back to his penis and alternate swirling, flicking, and sucking.

Don't take his penis too far into your mouth or you won't be able to pull off the suction

If you can't make him erect, create a usable erection by combining a hand trick with the female superior position. No matter what position he was in when he lost the erection, get on top now that it's gone. The visual stimulation of watching you ride him will excite and cause him to become erect once again.

Technique Tip

RIDING HIM HOME

Straddle him. Grasp the base of his penis firmly in one hand—as if you were going to give him a hand job.

Use the head of his penis to stroke and stimulate your genitals. When you are ready, lower your body onto his penis without letting go of the base in your hand.

If you have a good PC muscle—important in this technique!—grasp the first third of his penis, using your own muscle to simulate thrusting.

Should he remain flaccid, lean forward, supporting yourself on one hand resting beside his body, and work his penis up and down—also using your PC muscle at the same time—to bring yourself to orgasm. Alternate thrusting with the head stroke: using the head of his penis to stimulate your clitoris.

Whether or not he comes along for the ride, you'll get where you want to go.

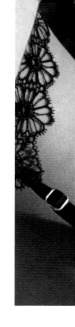

THE SEXUAL EPIPHANY

Create—or Sustain— a Sexual Epiphany

What is a sexual epiphany?

It is an erotic tsunami, not merely a nice day at the beach. When the physical and the spiritual elements of lovemaking come together in an *explosive* breakthrough experience that leaves you more solidly connected to each other—and deliriously happy—you've had a sexual epiphany. So much greater than *good* sex, epiphany sex takes you higher, to a new level of intimacy. The trick is getting there again.

But how will you know if you've had a sexual epiphany?

Here are the signs:

- You come away from the experience a little shaken—really, you or your lover may be trembling postorgasm—and/or

- You feel so deeply touched that you (or your lover) may cry or at least have tears in your eyes.

- On the other hand, you (or your lover) may be so exhilarated and exuberant that you're laughing out loud.

And you're suddenly more confident in your sexual abilities. You shed the last vestiges of body inhibitions. His performance anxiety disappeared. Effortlessly, you surmounted obstacles such as fatigue or irritation with each other.

And now something has changed inside you and inside the relationship. You feel the difference even if you can't express it in words.

Sexual epiphanies usually occur when sex is combined with a dramatic life event or a strong emotion that increases passion. You can get some mileage out of an epiphany without doing anything to help it along. But if you put a little effort into increasing the novelty and drama in your sex life, you can get much more from this one great experience.

The following are some epiphanies and the tactics for keeping them working their magic long after the bed has stopped shaking.

"Real talk"

"Throwing out birth control was like embarking on a journey together. The first night we made love to make a baby we were overcome by the depth of our feelings for each other. We seemed to melt into each other, we were so close," says Maya.

Her husband, Rick, adds, "The intensity of my feelings for her were overwhelming. It's as if we graduated to a new level of sexual intimacy and commitment."

THE SEXUAL EPIPHANY: BABY-MAKING SEX

Baby-making sex unleashes a heady mix of emotions. Your commitment to each other gets stronger. In a way, you are renewing your marriage vows. Suddenly every move you make in bed seems more meaningful because this could be the night that you create life.

This is a vulnerable time in a couple's life. Feelings are exposed, defenses are down. They are in a deeply trusting state and really connect with each other now. The timing is right for a sexual epiphany whether or not conception occurs .

The epiphany's calling card: *overwhelming tenderness.*

Your new closeness and stronger commitment make you exquisitely tender with each other. Skin is more sensitive to each other's touch. You both crave long kisses.

How to keep that epiphany working in your sex life: deep, slow lovemaking in a position that promotes eye contact and hands free for sensuous stroking.

The technique: *side by side intercourse.*

In the basic version, lie side by side facing each other. One puts a leg over the other. Move slowly and stroke, kiss, and fondle each other. Shift into one of the basic "on top" positions (affording deeper penetration) for the climax.

Variation: *the scissors position.*

He lies on his right side, while you lie next to him on your back, facing him, your right leg between his thighs and left leg on top of his left leg. (Make an X with your legs!) Even your legs caress in this position. (See page 108 for more on the side by side position.)

THE SEXUAL EPIPHANY: POST-TRAUMA SEX

You've been through a major trauma—for example, a severe case of postpartum depression, the death of a family member or close friend, getting fired, a cancer scare, an affair or serious emotional involvement with a "friend" of the opposite sex. Couples who overcome an infidelity often report having intense sexual epiphanies that bring them back together.

Traumas drain sexual energy. They leave you feeling too hurt to be touched. Then—pow!—all that pent-up and suppressed desire breaks out. You come together physically hungry and emotionally needy for each other.

The epiphany's calling card: *hard, hot, fast sex.*

Fueled in part by anger, fear, frustration, or grief, you go after each other like actors in a steamy film. Your hands move quickly up and down each other's bodies, as if they can't linger long on one hot patch of skin. This is the kind of sex that leaves you drenched and panting—and emotionally cleansed.

How to keep that epiphany working in your sex life: Maintain high speed.

The technique: *planned quickies.*

Quickies are brief episodes of lovemaking centered on intercourse, with only as much foreplay as it takes to get you both highly aroused. That's exactly how this epiphany played out. But quickies can be arranged.

Plan for a quickie: Fantasize the encounter in advance and grab bits of "foreplay" when you can. Run your hand suggestively down his chest or caress her butt as you're walking past each other in the hallway. Grab him for a hot kiss while you're clearing the dishes. Take small opportunities to caress and fondle each other. And wear clothing, such as a skirt, no panties, or a loose shirt, no bra, that makes you accessible to his touch. Use smoldering eye contact to encourage those touches.

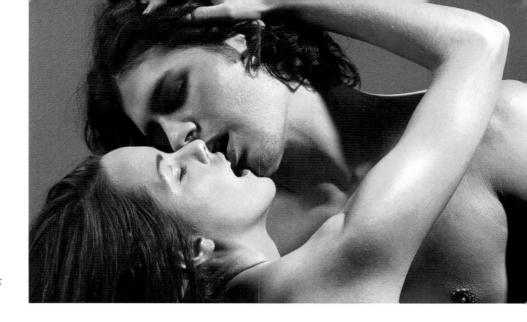

THE SEXUAL EPIPHANY: REDISCOVERY SEX

Nothing is "wrong," but you're not having frequent, satisfying sex. "No time, no energy" has become your mantra. You catch each other's eyes at a party—and suddenly you're hot for each other again. Shyly, with hearts pounding, you make your way back together.

The epiphany's calling card: *awkward sex that quickly turns into the surest moves you've ever made.*

You bump noses when you come together for that first deep kiss in a long time. He fumbles with your hooks. Your hands shake on his zipper. Then you touch skin. The awkwardness dissipates in the heat of the most intense desire you've ever felt.

How to keep that epiphany working in your sex life: Create erotic fantasies together.

The technique: *Fantasy Encounters.*

Keep sex on your mind. Carole Pasahow, D.S.W., created the 21-Day Passion Fix program for couples who have been ignoring or repressing their sexual thoughts and urges. Fantasy Encounters, mental foreplay you do together, are key to the plan.

Set aside thirty minutes of quiet time one night a week. Create a fantasy that you will both use as your "arousal story" that week. (You may act it out in full or in part—or you may simply each fantasize the story before sex.) Develop a sexually detailed story that is mutually exciting. For example, you might create a tale of sex in an exotic locale or a different time period or one of you might be a love slave to the other. Be creative! (See pages 233.)

"Real talk"

"We were in that no-sex rut," says Lydia. "Except for the good-night kiss and an occasional hug, we were barely touching. My mom was in town visiting, so we went to 'our bar' for a drink. I saw a couple touching each other's hands and arms the way we used to do and my eyes filled with tears. I wanted that, too! He looked at me and read my mind. We went home and had sex in the shower so Mom and the kids wouldn't hear us. It was the most intense, exhilarating experience. We couldn't stop laughing afterward."

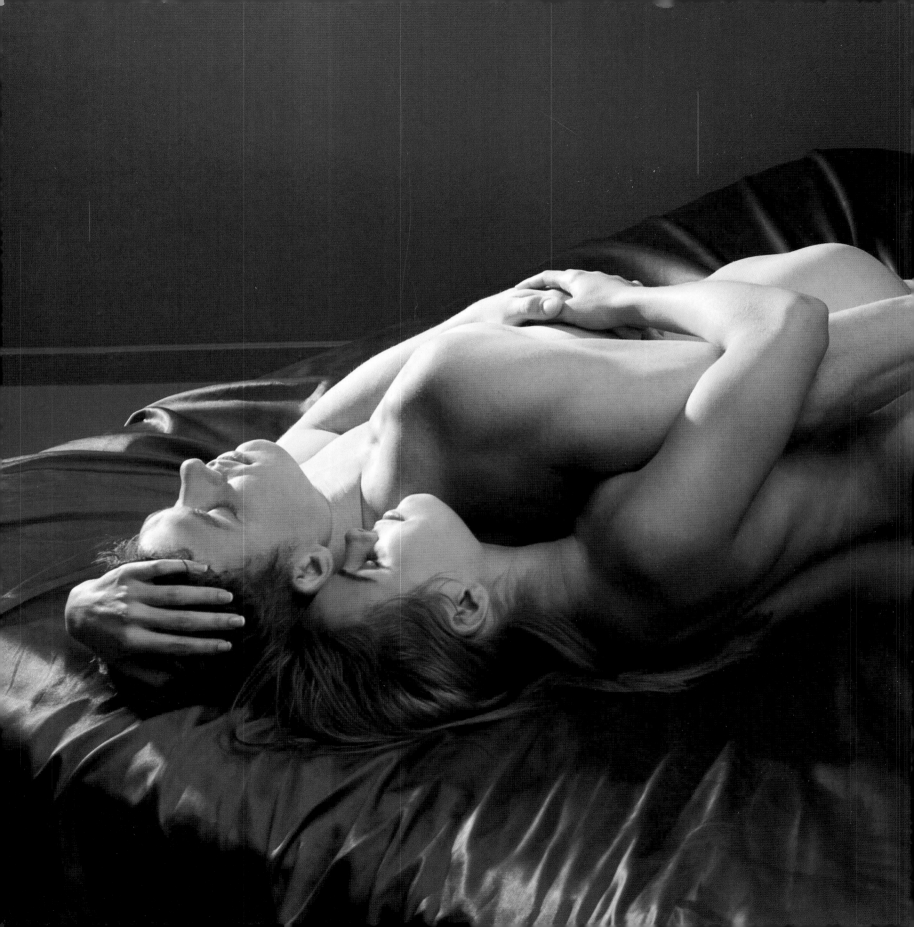